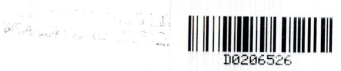

Being a Cancer Patient's Carer

A guide

Wesley C Finegan

MB BCh BAO MRCGP MICGP D Pall Med

Radcliffe Publishing

Oxford • Seattle

Radcliffe Publishing Ltd
18 Marcham Road
Abingdon
Oxon OX14 1AA
United Kingdom

www.radcliffe-oxford.com
Electronic catalogue and worldwide online ordering facility.

British Library Cataloguing in Publication Data

A catalogue record for this book is available from the British Library.

ISBN 1 85775 638 X

Typeset by Anne Joshua & Associates, Oxford
Printed and bound by TJ International Ltd, Padstow, Cornwall

Contents

About the author

I was aged three when I first announced that I wanted to be a doctor. In 1978 I achieved that aim when I qualified from The Queen's University of Belfast. After a further four years of training, I entered general practice in east Sussex.

In 1976 I met Alice and we were married in 1979. We have two children, Chris and Sharon.

While working in general practice, I developed an increasing interest in caring for patients with cancer and this led to me being appointed as a consultant in palliative medicine in central Scotland in 1991.

In 1994 I became a cancer patient myself and had to retire from my hospice post on the grounds of ill health. I was very fortunate to be offered a post with the University of Dundee where I continue to offer some input into their courses on cancer and palliative care.

Last year I had another recurrence of my cancer. A month after completing treatment, Alice also developed cancer. As her carer, I have not needed to use many of the skills I learned at medical school but I did realise how useful it was to have my specialist knowledge and know what to ask and whom. Caring for each other has taught us a lot and we have thought about many things that we never had to consider before.

Hopefully, by sharing some of the things Alice and I have learned while caring for each other, we can make your role as carer a little easier.

Wesley C Finegan
November 2004

Acknowledgements

I would like to thank my wife Alice, who taught me so much about being a carer both when she was caring for me and latterly when I became her carer.

I acknowledge, with gratitude, the help and advice offered by Patricia Manson BDS in her comments on the chapters on coping with a dry mouth and coping with a sore mouth.

I also wish to thank all the people who taught me so much about caring – especially my patients and their families.

Finally I thank the staff at Radcliffe Publishing, who have advised me and helped me throughout the producing of this book.

Introduction

It is estimated that one in eight people are carers, but not all of these people are caring for cancer patients. Because the relationship between carer and patient is so varied, including family, professional carers, friends and lay carers, the term 'the patient' has been chosen as the most universally applicable wording to cover the various relationships between the carer and the person being cared for.

This book is primarily written for the non-professional carer and is intended to offer practical advice and ideas. Many of the topics are also covered from a slightly different perspective in the companion volume *Trust Me, I'm a ~~Doctor~~ Cancer Patient* (Radcliffe Medical Press, 2004. ISBN 1 85775 877 3). This is unavoidable since both books need to be free-standing and not dependent on each other.

How do you use this book?

I have been a cancer patient for ten years and more recently I have cared for my wife Alice, who also has cancer. I have been increasingly aware of the need for patients, doctors, nurses and other carers to work together to achieve realistic and achievable goals. That's why I wrote this book.

As a child, I once saw a bicycle with two riders. I asked my mother about it and she explained that it was a 'tandem'. She explained how one person steered but both shared the work of pedalling. I have used the same idea in this book and in the companion volume *Trust Me, I'm a ~~Doctor~~ Cancer Patient*. I'll try and steer you through the maze of decisions and practical problems you and the patient will face, always with the concept of working 'in tandem' with the doctors and nurses who are looking after the patient.

How can you all work 'in tandem'? The word 'tandem' is used in the chapters to break the problem into six sections to make it easier for you to find the information you need. The TANDEM acronym breaks each of the chapters into the following sections.

The doctor says

Here I will give you some relevant information to help you understand more about the problem being discussed.

We then use the word TANDEM to examine the various issues from different aspects.

T Think

You are facing new situations regularly as a carer. Hopefully I can help you think through the issues you might have to face.

A Ask

There is so much to learn. Where does one start? What do you need to know and who can tell you the answers? I'll try and help you with some of the questions I have asked.

N Note

Making a note of a relevant detail now might save you a lot of difficulty remembering those elusive facts in a few weeks' time!

D Do ✓

Here I will offer you some practical ideas that have been tried and tested by my patients and some that worked for Alice and me.

E Explore

Sometimes we want to know more or find out about something we would like to know about. I'll try and guide you to the best sources of information.

M More Information

If there is something that has not been said already and it's relevant, you'll find it here.

Throughout the text I assume that you have no specialist training as this is often the case where family members and others take responsibility for daily care. For this reason, you will be advised to seek advice from a professional carer but I do recognise that some readers will have the necessary skills and knowledge to make their own decisions.

To appeal to as wide a readership as possible, I refer to 'the patient' because you might not necessarily be a family member, although this will often be the case. Where the word 'relative' is used, this can mean a spouse, partner or any family member.

Dedication

This book is dedicated to the following people:

- our children, Chris and Sharon, who have coped so well with our illnesses, helping us to continue having a normal family life and maintain a sense of perspective throughout
- our longstanding friends David and Brenda, for their unfailing support and help
- the many other friends and relatives who have helped us in so many ways
- the various doctors and nurses who have cared for us through difficult and challenging times.

Preparing to be a Carer

Chapter 1

On becoming a carer

Knowing is not enough; we must apply
Willing is not enough: we must do.

Goethe

Time to make plans, promises and pledges

It is likely, if you are reading this, that you have accepted responsibility for caring for a relative or friend who has cancer. Obviously there will be some issues discussed in this book that will not be relevant to your patient, so please don't feel obliged to read every page. Because the relationship between the carer and the sufferer can be so varied, I will use the term 'patient', rather than assume that it is a relative you are caring for.

I am not writing a manual explaining 'how to do it'. I am sharing some thoughts, based on my own experience as a doctor who specialised in the care of patients with advanced cancer, as a cancer patient myself for over ten years and more recently as a carer for my wife, Alice, who has also been treated for cancer.

One of the easiest 'traps' to fall into is to feel obliged to promise just about anything when you care for a patient who has cancer. Let me say now that this is a common reaction, but you can't always make promises at the time because you simply don't know what is ahead of you and the patient. Don't be afraid to agree to *plan* to be there and continue to care, but to allow yourself limits to what you can realistically offer. Your circumstances might change. A *promise* is much more binding than an agreement or *plan* to give as much input as possible.

So, plan, don't promise!

Here are some of the things you need to think about when you become a carer.

- The patient's mobility and independence – e.g. to get to the bathroom.
- The patient's ability to wash/dress and make simple meals.
- The patient's ability to be left alone and for how long.
- The patient's ability to be responsible for their medication.
- The patient's need for transport to hospital or clinic appointments and how often this need arises. Can you take the patient to the appointments or is a driver required?
- The financial implications.

In the early days, some of these questions will be very hard to answer accurately and the best response may be an 'educated guess'.

Can you take some time off work? Alice took unpaid leave to look after me. Her employer was very sympathetic to our needs and allowed her to work part-time for a while to care for me. Obviously you won't earn as much if you work part-time, but in the interim, while you make longer-term plans, it might be an option.

No time to plan – the diagnosis was so sudden

The diagnosis of cancer almost always comes as a shock, even when patients have been unwell for some time. When cancer is diagnosed after a short illness one can suddenly be plunged into a new role as the carer, with little or no time to prepare.

This is what happened to Alice and me. I had just completed a month-long course of treatment for a recurrence of my cancer. Alice had been vaguely unwell for a couple of weeks but had assumed that she was suffering from the 'bug' that was affecting about half of the workforce at the hospital where she worked.

Alice had planned to have a few days off and on the first of these days (a Wednesday) we were going to see friends for coffee. Alice awoke feeling unwell and told me she didn't think she could make the half-hour journey. I examined her and was unhappy with my findings.

Hearing bad news is not easy. Giving it is not easy either, but telling my wife that I thought she might have cancer was the hardest thing I've ever had to do. Alice was fortunate enough to be able to see the doctor that morning in a cancelled appointment and Alice spent our planned three days off having X-rays and various other tests. On Monday we had the diagnosis confirmed.

In one sense it was easy for us. I was already off work due to my illness and I was well enough to drive short distances. I had plenty of spare time so I was able to care for Alice, just as she had done when I was first diagnosed and she was at home with our young children. We were also fortunate in that Alice's work was only ten minutes from home and she could pop home at lunchtime and see that I was OK when I was having treatment.

A sudden diagnosis can bring many unforeseen changes to your carefully made plans. We had to cancel three planned holidays and short breaks including our silver wedding anniversary celebration.

Our daughter was getting married and everything was planned and arranged when Alice was diagnosed with cancer three months before the 'big day'. We discussed deferring the date and decided to leave things as they were. Our basis for this was that we estimated that Alice would be having chemotherapy and we could adjust the treatment dates if necessary so that Alice was 'at her best' between treatments. Setting a new date (if we could get one) could bring new unknowns to face. As it happened, on the date we did think about, I was in hospital having chemotherapy for a recurrence of my cancer!

The wedding went well, Alice coped well with the busy weeks before the wedding and the day itself and very few people were aware that she had lost her hair and was wearing a wig, even when she removed her traditional 'mother of the bride hat'!

Looking back, if we had been given more warning, we might have tried to change our plans. It probably worked out for the best that we simply kept to our original arrangements.

It's not always as easy as this, so what can you do?

We had lots of offers of help, some of which we didn't need, but we quickly learned that when people offer to help, it's because they want to and there was almost always something that we could gratefully accept. Sometimes it was a lift to a distant hospital for an appointment or sometimes it was more basic, like getting shopping when we were less fit to carry heavy bags. Don't refuse any offer; you might not need it just now, but sooner or later you might be glad of the help!

Reacting to the news

How are you likely to react to hearing unexpected bad news like this? Here are some relatively common responses to hearing that the patient has cancer.

- Anger – because you see yourself being robbed of your free time or a future together.
- Denial – the patient looks far too well to be so seriously ill. It's a mistake.
- Disbelief – it can't be true when the patient seems so well.
- Fear – what will happen next?

Facing new challenges

You do not have to be endowed with any special skills to be a carer. If you can make a hot drink, fix the pillows, open or close a window or help the patient get into and out of a chair, that's a good start. I used very few of my medical skills in looking after Alice.

You'll almost certainly face new situations as a carer. There will be things to be done that you've never done before. You'll learn new skills as you go along. Don't look at the professional nurses and feel inadequate. They were like you once – facing a new task for the first time – but they have spent years training and repeatedly doing their job. You can, and will, develop new skills, and the professional carers will advise and help you.

Your support, company and encouragement will all help the patient as they face new and challenging situations.

You and the patient need to agree what input and practical care you can offer and what they can accept. It may be inappropriate for you to be expected to offer intimate care. I recall looking after a lady and assuming that her husband could help her wash and dress. Even after over 40 years of marriage she found this unacceptable and the good man sat reading his paper while the community nurses helped his wife wash and dress. Similarly, an evening visit was required to get her to bed.

You and the patient must agree about your role and make sure that someone else takes responsibility for any aspect of care that you cannot undertake. Nobody will mind, nobody will be critical of your feelings and decisions. We all have our boundaries and patients have a right to their privacy.

Encourage the patient to explore new opportunities, e.g. using their enforced free time to explore a new hobby, finish that book they started years before, or finish something that they started that is a realistic and achievable goal that will give them some pleasure.

Need to know more?

I must remind you that the doctors, nurses and other healthcare professionals have a duty to respect the privacy and confidentiality of their patients. This means that they will not discuss the patient's problems or treatment with you without the patient giving their consent each time a discussion is requested. This in no way undermines or fails to recognise your input – it is simply the code of ethical practice under which the various healthcare professionals work and breach of this rule of confidentiality can carry serious consequences for them.

Further reading

Lee E (2002) *In Your Own Time*. Oxford University Press, Oxford.

Chapter 2

BEFRIENDing the patient

Don't walk in front of me; I may not follow. Don't walk behind me; I may not lead.
Walk beside me and just be my friend.

Albert Camus

As we discussed in Chapter 1, it is perfectly normal for patients and their carers to agree what the carer's input should be. Equally, as a carer, you are not expected to be a trained healthcare professional. Most of my specialist skills were not necessary in caring for Alice. It is possible that there will be duties that you don't feel able to undertake, but there is one thing we all can be – a friend to the sick person.

To give the patient our best care, we need to BEFRIEND them. The word 'befriend' is my reminder to think about the patient's Beliefs, Education, Family, Religion, Infection risk, Expectations, Nutrition and Difficulties they are experiencing.

I have included a few examples under each of these categories to illustrate the variety of ways in which almost anyone can help the patient. I am sure you'll be able to add many more of your own.

B Beliefs

- Cultural
- Personal
- Religious

Do your personal and religious beliefs or cultural traditions agree with those of the person you are looking after? The nurses popping in and out may be unaware of a patient's personal beliefs. If you are there all day, you may find it necessary to discuss their religious needs and even find out more about how to accommodate these needs into your caring routine. For example, are you aware of the importance and implications of religious feasts and fasts, e.g. Ramadan? In some cultures, the position of the bed is very important. If the patient is staying with you, these may be very important issues for them. This is discussed further in Chapter 38.

E Education

- About the illness
- About the treatment
- About the probable prognosis

How much do you know about the patient's illness, treatment and the likely outcome? Who gave you the information? Can you be sure it is accurate? How much does the patient know? (Not what do they *think* they know!) I believe it is easiest if you and the patient can honestly share the information about their illness and use it to set realistic goals that you can achieve together.

Having said this, the patient has the right not to let you know what is going on and the staff cannot divulge information without his or her consent.

F Family

- Do your values and beliefs conflict with those of the patient?
- Consent – is there agreement over who gives consent to treatment if the patient is under age or has impaired understanding? How do you resolve these disagreements?
- How are other members of the family coping with their relative's illness?

The use of the word 'relative' in this book should be interpreted in the wider context and does not only mean the 'nuclear family'. As carers, we need to see beyond minor differences of opinion and respect the views and wishes of the patient. This can be difficult, and sometimes one has to agree to differ over what is deemed to be the best course of action.

If you are looking after a young person or someone who is not competent to make their own decisions about treatment, it is essential to involve all the relevant family members in the process of making the decisions about treatment, etc.

If you are the main carer, are the family members all fully aware of the patient's condition? How well are they coping? Could they offer more help or are they overwhelmed?

R Religion

- Are there any issues that affect acceptance of treatment – e.g. Jehovah's Witness and blood transfusion? What about compliance with medications during Ramadan, when one cannot eat or drink anything (including medications) from dawn to sunset?
- Do the patient's religious beliefs affect how they view their illness in terms of acceptance of the illness, prognosis and/or treatment?

There are far too many religious and cultural issues for me to deal with in this book. The two quoted above are really issues that need to be addressed by the professionals, but it is important for you to discuss these issues with the patient. If necessary, ask them for guidance so that you do not cause them offence or avoidable distress by inadvertently breaking a religious rule or moral code. For further discussion *see* Chapter 38.

I Infection risk

- Has your fear of picking up an infection resulted in the patient not getting appropriate care?

Cancer is not an infectious illness. You probably know that, but some people don't. Cancer cannot be passed to another person by touching, kissing or sexual contact.

What is important to remember is that while receiving chemotherapy, patients are much more prone to infections. If a visitor has an infectious illness, keep them at bay until they are fully recovered!

Patients suffering from HIV/AIDS can develop cancer. There is no major risk to you as a carer if you take adequate precautions to protect yourself from exposure to body fluids. Gloves are usually sufficient and it is likely that there will be nurses in attendance who will be able to instruct you in how to take adequate precautions to protect yourself from infection risk.

E Expectations

- Are the patient's past experiences affecting present/future expectations?
- Are the anticipated outcome of the present illness and the expectation of the future realistic?

You need to think about these questions from your own perspective and that of your patient.

Who gave you the information on which you are basing your expectations of the outcome of the illness? Is the source reliable, accurate and dependable?

Does your expectation agree with that of the patient? If not, ask yourself why. Does someone need to discuss this with the patient and make them aware of the facts? The patient might have personal business they need to attend to and may have less time than they had thought.

N Nutrition

- What are the effects of the illness or treatment on the patient's nutritional state? Is there any loss of appetite?
- Are cultural dietary needs being met? Is the appropriate ethnic diet available?
- Think about foods, and religious fasts e.g. Yom Kippur.

Most patients experience some loss of appetite (*see* Chapter 12) when having chemotherapy, but on the other hand, treatment with steroids can make one feel hungry all the time.

If the patient follows a religion that you are not familiar with, find out about feasts and fasts. The laws concerning these practices must be strictly adhered to and you could cause offence by failing to recognise the strict rules that govern such special days. Some further information is included in Chapter 38.

D Difficulties

- Difficulty getting to hospital appointments
- Problems with daily life
- Unpleasant or painful symptoms and associated problems

- Communication problems – sensory impairment/speech difficulty
- Not fluent in your language
- Learning disability

Patients receiving treatment often are too unwell to drive themselves to hospital or clinic appointments. Public transport is not a realistic option if one has to change buses or trains and hospital transport is busy and one almost always seems to go 'round the world' while other patients are collected or left home. Prolonging one's journey when feeling sick and tired is not an option one chooses readily.

If you can drive and have the time, you can provide a very valuable and much appreciated service.

Similarly, simple gestures such as a meal ready to heat and eat or freshly made meals ready to freeze and eat later are always appreciated. Friends of ours did this for us when Alice was ill and it was something we appreciated very much. Apart from the convenience, one knows that it's good food and not full of preservatives and unwanted additives. You don't need special training to offer this kind of help.

Most cancer patients will experience some pain or other symptoms. Some of the common ones are discussed in Section 3 of this book – 'Practical problems'.

Sometimes family members are the best equipped to cope with an ongoing existing communication problem. If loss of speech is a new problem, don't forget that the patient can still hear you! A notebook might help them and allow them to write down what they wish to say, but you can reply in the usual way.

Deafness can often be overcome by writing notes.

If the patient does not speak the same language as yourself, you face a problem! Thankfully this does not happen very often!

Learning disabled patients can have difficulty expressing pain or other problems. Often the person who has looked after them and known them longest can interpret their behaviour and have a pretty good understanding of the problem. Don't be afraid to ask!

Chapter 3

Taking time for yourself

The doctor says

When you are very busy looking after a sick patient, it's very easy to neglect yourself and forget to take time for your own health and wellbeing.

Don't feel guilty for asking someone else to take over and give you a day off or accepting the offer of a respite admission to the hospice or nursing home.

If you are offered such a break, don't feel obliged to visit every day as many people do. Have a break. Go away for a few days, have a hair-do, a manicure, a meal out with friends or whatever allows you to relax and unwind. The whole idea is that you return refreshed and ready to resume your responsibilities.

Dealing with serious illness in a relative or close friend can make us become very aware of our own health. It's natural for us to stop and reflect on how suddenly things have changed for the patient and to wonder if we could also have some undiagnosed illness waiting to manifest itself. This is discussed further in Chapter 4.

Think

- When did you last have a break?
- Is the patient's condition reasonably stable at present? It is always best to try and have a break when the patient's illness seems to be reasonably stable. Things can change suddenly but this is not a reason for you to feel guilty for taking a much-needed break.
- Think about where the patient could be admitted for respite and start making enquiries about available dates, etc.

Ask

- Ask the patient how they feel about your need for a short break. Patients sometimes feel threatened by the carer's need for a holiday, wondering how they will be cared for. If the patient is apprehensive, it might be possible to arrange a visit to the hospice or nursing home where they could go for respite. This might allay their fears.
- Ask the doctor, social worker or specialist nurse about suitable places for respite admissions. Many local health authorities have lists of local nursing homes, which are available on request.

Note

- Make a note of any special needs the patient has. If they require special nursing care or have specific nursing needs, make sure these can be provided.
- Make a note of all medications to be given, the times and doses. If there are any injections or special treatments that are given by the nurse, make sure the staff know about these and which nurse to contact if there are any queries.
- After a first visit or admission, make a note of any aspects of care that were especially good or of any issues that need to be addressed on a subsequent admission. In fairness, many of the 'problems' that one faces are associated with getting used to new routines and policies and these are often much less of a problem on a second admission. We all do things better second time around!

Do ☑

- Make sure that you leave your contact details and itinerary with the staff of the hospice or nursing home.
- Tell the nurses and doctor of the dates and venue of any respite admissions planned.
- Order adequate supplies of all the medications the patient needs to cover the entire time of the admission.
- If you are going abroad and your return could possibly be delayed, make sure that you have negotiated a longer admission for care and have ordered enough extra tablets to cover this possibility.
- Leave clear instructions or have someone available to act on your behalf in the event of an unforeseen development.

Explore

- It might not be appropriate for you to go away for a holiday or a break at this time. Perhaps day care would be appropriate on a regular basis, allowing you to get out to do the shopping, have a day to yourself or simply take time to meet a friend for a cup of coffee.
- Take time to explore the various options available. Talk to the nurse, social worker or doctor and see what is available in your area.

More Information

Looking after a patient with cancer often makes us think about how things could have been if the disease had been detected earlier or if it could possibly have been prevented.

There are many factors associated with the development of cancer. These include:

- exposure to pollutants – smoking, industrial fumes and chemicals
- your individual genetic make-up. Some cancers affect several members of the same family.

It is pointless to sit blaming ourselves for what has happened, but it can be helpful to know a bit more about the warning signs for some of the commoner cancers, so I've listed some facts about some common cancers in the next chapter, 'Thinking about your own health'.

Chapter 4

Thinking about your own health

The doctor says

It's very easy to become so involved with caring for the patient that you can neglect your own health. The check-up with the dentist, the mammogram or smear test you were due to have or even a simple blood pressure check can all become consigned to the increasing list of things to do 'when you have time'.

Let me remind you that you are important too, which you can so easily forget. Try and find someone who can allow you to keep that appointment. Getting a clean bill of health will give you peace of mind but, if anything is wrong, it is always best that it is caught early on. Here I can speak from personal experience – my wife was busy looking after me while I had treatment for a recurrence of my cancer. It transpired that she too had cancer even though she had no symptoms at the time. That's why your doctor offers 'screening clinics' – to pick up the people who look well and feel well but have disease at an early, detectable and treatable stage.

Think

Cancer is not an infectious disease. You won't catch cancer by looking after the patient, but you might have been wondering why several members of your family have had the same or a similar cancer.

- Has anyone else in your family had cancer?
- If so, think about who had cancer and what kind of cancer, if you know this.
- Are you worried about developing cancer later in your own life?

The American Cancer Society offered a simple seven-point checklist some 20 years ago – 1983 to be precise. It advised 'CAUTION':

C Change in bladder or bowel habit
A Any sore or wound that does not heal
U Unusual bleeding or a discharge
T Thickening or a lump in a breast or the testicle or elsewhere
I Indigestion or difficulty in swallowing
O Obvious change in a mole or wart (change in size or behaviour – itch or bleeding)
N Nagging cough or persisting hoarseness

If you are suffering from any of these, consult your doctor – now.

Ask

If you are anxious about your own risk of developing cancer, it might help for you to discuss this with your doctor. There are a number of things we all can do to try and reduce our risk of developing cancer – stop smoking (or don't start), drink alcohol in moderation, eat a balanced diet, take regular exercise and attend for screening tests like regular smears.

You'll find more details about a number of commoner cancers in the 'More Information' section.

Note

Make a note of the reasons why you think that you might be at risk of developing cancer. If you have a persisting symptom like the ones listed in the 'More Information' section below, make a note of it and see your doctor for advice without undue delay.

Sometimes it is helpful to make a note of which members of your family have had cancer and what kind of cancer they had. What is most important is to note any blood relatives who have been affected by similar types of cancer. For example, two sisters, or several generations in one family having breast cancer could indicate a genetic risk for the female children.

Sometimes it can be hard to accurately compile this kind of information. Our older relatives did not speak about cancer as freely as we do today.

Do

Attend for any screening tests or clinics offered to you. Disease caught at an early stage is always easier to manage and has a better chance of being treated successfully.

Fear and embarrassment are common reasons for people putting off attending the doctor even when they are worried. Try to overcome these and go and be seen.

The absence of pain in a swelling or lump does not mean that it is safe to ignore. Most cancers are painless in the early stages. If in doubt, go and see the doctor – now.

Explore

Information about cancer, especially the treatments available, is constantly being updated and it can take quite a long time before an author writes an update and gets it published in a book. For this reason, Internet websites are the most up to date.

The CancerBACUP website www.cancerbacup.org.uk is very easy to use and is regularly updated. Another website that is user friendly is www.irishhealth.com which is based in Ireland and may be of particular interest to readers living in that country. The information found on these websites is checked and approved by qualified professionals. Be very careful when you do explore any topic related to healthcare that it has been written by suitably qualified people.

More Information 📖

Here is some very basic and brief information about some of the commoner cancers. Space only allows the briefest discussion about these, so you might want to look at other sources of information such as websites or a book in your local library.

Please note that the symptoms in the following lists are not in order of importance or significance.

Almost all cancers are commoner in smokers and those who drink more than the recommended amounts of alcohol, but just because you don't smoke and don't drink excessive amounts of alcohol does not mean you can't develop cancer. My wife and are both life-long non-smokers with a very low alcohol intake and are both cancer patients.

In general, any unexplained loss of weight or a symptom that does not settle within the time frame when you'd expect it to improve should be investigated. I have broken the lists into groups to help you find the ones that might be relevant to you. I could not possibly include every possible early sign of all the cancers, so the message is 'if in doubt, ask the doctor'.

Cancers affecting men and women

- Bladder and kidney
- Colorectal
- Larynx
- Lung
- Lymphomas
- Mouth
- Stomach and upper bowel

Bladder and kidney

Kidney cancer affects men more commonly than women. Bladder cancer is sometimes associated with exposure to certain industrial chemicals, including aniline dyes.

Report any of these symptoms to your doctor:

- blood in your urine
- pain or difficulty passing urine
- persisting pain in your side
- tiredness and anaemia
- weight loss.

Colorectal

The lining of our bowel is constantly being renewed, so the cells are very active and minor abnormalities can occur and result in benign polyps and other growths. Some of these will become cancerous, so any symptoms are worth checking out. Here are the ones you should look out for and report:

- a change in your bowel habit persisting for four weeks or more
- anaemia discovered on routine testing but with no specific cause identified
- persistent bleeding – more than four weeks.

Do not assume that bleeding is due to haemorrhoids. While any of these symptoms can be due to benign causes, putting off the checks is only increasing the risk that disease could be advanced by the time it is diagnosed.

Larynx

The larynx is that part of your throat where your voice comes from. Cancers of the larynx are commoner in smokers and heavy drinkers. Report any of the following symptoms to your doctor:

- blood in your phlegm (sputum)
- hoarseness persisting more than one week
- the sensation of a lump in your throat.

Lung

I hardly need to remind you that lung cancer is associated with smoking. It is possible that you are less aware that it can also be associated with exposure to industrial dust of various kinds and, of course, there is a specific lung tumour associated with asbestos exposure. Exposure to asbestos does not have to be prolonged, as is often believed. Report to your doctor if any of these apply to you:

- chest pain
- cough – a new cough persisting for more than one month, or a change in the pattern of a cough you have had for a long time
- coughing up blood
- recurring chest infections which you have not suffered from before
- shortness of breath.

Lymphomas

The lymphomas are a group of cancers that are broadly broken down into Hodgkin's lymphoma (sometimes referred to as 'Hodgkin's disease') and non-Hodgkin's lymphoma. They can affect young and older people. The symptoms include the following, which should be reported to your doctor:

- a lump, often in the neck or other lymph glands
- alcohol intolerance – abdominal pain or chest pain (sometimes)
- fever – no obvious reason
- itching, sometimes quite intense and which may come and go
- night sweats.

Mouth

Mouth cancer is commoner in people over the age of 50, but can affect any age group, so don't assume that you are too young. The things to report include:

- a persisting sore mouth or sore throat
- an ulcer or a sore area that does not heal after three weeks
- any lump or thickened area in your mouth
- any red or white patch.

Stomach and upper bowel

Cancer of the stomach is commoner in people who have had previous surgery to the stomach, eat an excess of smoked or spicy food, or smoke and drink heavily.
   The symptoms to look out for and report include:

- blood in your motions (usually dark brown or black)
- difficulty in swallowing
- indigestion
- loss of appetite
- loss of weight
- pain in your upper abdomen.

Cancers affecting women

- Breast
- Cervix
- Ovary

Breast

Become 'Breast Aware'. Take time to look after yourself using this five-point plan. Breast cancer is much less common in men, but it can occur.

- Know what changes to look and feel for.
- Know what is normal for you.
- Look and feel regularly (at least once a month).
- Report any changes to your doctor without delay (e.g. a lump, a retracted nipple, a discharge from the nipple, 'eczema' or a rash round your nipple or any change in shape or size of one breast).
- If you are offered a breast screening appointment (mammogram), do attend.

Cervix (the neck of the womb)

Several factors affect your risk of developing cancer of the cervix. These include an early start to your sexual activity, multiple sexual partners, long-term use of the pill and cigarette smoking.
   Cervical cancer is often detected at an early, treatable stage by screening, so do attend for regular smears.

Ask your doctor for advice if you have any of the following symptoms:

- bleeding after intercourse
- irregular bleeding (in post-menopausal women this may be due to cancer of the womb, as well as cancer of the cervix)
- vaginal discharge, usually blood stained, sometimes smelly.

Ovary

Cancer of the ovary is one of those cancers that can be very hard to detect because the ovary can grow to quite a size before it causes any symptoms. At present there is no satisfactory test that can be easily offered to the general population, but if there is a history of ovarian cancer in your family, it is worth bearing this in mind.

Ovarian cancer is commoner as one gets older, but any age can be affected. It tends to be commoner in women who have not had children.

Ask your doctor if you have:

- a feeling of fullness low in your abdomen
- irregular vaginal bleeding
- pain on sexual intercourse.

Cancers affecting men

- Prostate
- Testicle

Prostate

Prostate cancer can lie silent for a long time and by the time you develop symptoms, it can be quite advanced. For this reason, it is a very good idea to attend for screening tests and any 'well men' clinics that are offered by your doctor. When detected early, prostate cancer can be managed much more successfully. The things to report are:

- blood in your urine
- pain on passing urine
- persisting back pain
- slowness of your stream when passing urine – many older men experience slowness of their urinary stream as the gland enlarges, but don't assume it's just your age!

Testicle

This tumour tends to be commoner in younger men, with about 60% of tumours occurring in men aged 17–35 and 40% in those over 35, but all swellings of the testicle must be checked out. The risk of developing a cancerous tumour of the testicles is greater if you had an undescended testicle as a boy. Report to the doctor if you have:

- a lump in or around the testicle
- blood in the fluid when you ejaculate
- one testicle larger than the other
- pain in your testicles which does not settle after treatment
- swollen breasts (in young men). Men can get breast cancer too! Look at the notes about breast cancer in the list above to find out more. Men should always ask the doctor for advice if either or both breasts is persistently enlarged.

Further reading

Banks I (2004) *The Haynes Cancer Manual*. Haynes Publishing, Yeovil.
This is a practical step-by-step guide for men dealing with prevention, early detection and beating cancer.
Daniel R and Ellis R (2001) *The Cancer Prevention Book*. Simon and Schuster, London.
Rees GJF (2000) *The British Medical Association Family Doctor Guide to Cancer*. Dorling Kindersley, London.

Chapter 5

Taking responsibility for the patient's personal affairs

The doctor says

Cancer is a progressive illness and, sadly, the time will probably come when the patient will not be mobile enough or have the energy to take full responsibility for their personal affairs. It may be appropriate for you to discuss whether you should take on some of these responsibilities when the time is right. It can take some time to set up certain agreements such as power of attorney, so don't delay too long in making plans.

Think

How much responsibility you have depends on two basic factors:

- how much responsibility you want to take and
- how much the patient wishes you to do for them.

How much responsibility do you need to take on? Again this depends on two basic factors:

- Is the patient mentally capable of retaining control of their affairs?
- Is the patient mentally incapable of managing their affairs?

Ask

If the patient is mentally competent, you might wish to ask whether you should:

- collect benefits or pensions if these are not sent directly to their bank account
- set up a *third party mandate* that authorises you to operate the patient's bank account (this should not be used if the patient's mental state deteriorates).
- arrange a *power of attorney,* which gives you the legal right to manage the patient's affairs. A legal stationer can supply the document, but it is probably best for you to get a qualified solicitor to draw up the agreement. Power of attorney is valid while the patient is mentally capable of understanding what you are doing. In England and Wales, *enduring power of attorney* remains valid when the patient becomes mentally incapable of managing their own affairs, but the document giving power of attorney must have been signed when the patient was fully capable of understanding what they were agreeing to. If enduring power of attorney has not been arranged and the patient becomes mentally incapable of managing their affairs, it may be necessary to apply to the

Court of Protection for authorisation to manage the patient's finances. This is a costly and complicated procedure. If possible, try and arrange enduring power of attorney while the patient is capable of giving consent to this agreement.

In Scotland, a solicitor must draw up the power of attorney agreement and it remains valid if the patient subsequently becomes mentally incapable.

If the patient is mentally incapable of managing their own affairs, in England and Wales you could ask the Department for Work and Pensions about becoming the patient's *appointee*. This empowers you to claim and collect social security benefits on the patient's behalf and spend them on their needs.

In Scotland, a *curator bonis* is appointed by the court and in many cases the person appointed is a solicitor or accountant. The curator then manages all the financial and property affairs of the patient. This is an expensive process to set up and incurs an annual fee to cover administration costs.

Note

Make a note of the patient's wishes with respect to the management of their financial and personal affairs and the names of any professionals such as accountants and solicitors whose services the patient has previously used.

Do

If you are like me, you'll not like being responsible for someone else's money. The last thing you need is for someone to question how much is being spent. A few simple ideas can help save you from having to worry too much.

- Tell the patient what you are buying and show them the items.
- Keep receipts for everything you buy on the patient's behalf.
- Keep a simple account system showing what you spent the patient's money on and be prepared to show this to anyone who questions how much is being spent.

Explore

I have mentioned several organisations. If you wish to find out more and explore any of these further, here are some addresses.

- Citizens Advice Bureau – see your telephone directory for local office details.
- Court of Protection, Public Trust Office, Protection Division, Stewart House, 24 Kingsway, London WC2B 6JX.

More Information

The Carers National Association can offer advice and information to carers and Age Concern publishes a range of books and factsheets on various topics, including pensions. You should find these in your public library.

Chapter 6

Financial issues associated with being a carer

The doctor says

Caring for a patient with a serious and prolonged illness can be costly for you, the carer. You might have had to give up work or reduce the number of hours you work in order to provide the necessary care. The patient may be on a reduced salary or state benefit, which may be much less than your usual income.

Added to this there is the cost of visits to hospital and expenses that may be unforeseen, such as having to heat the house 24 hours a day when the heating was previously turned off when the house was empty during the working day.

Think

What is the cost of being a carer? Sometimes there are few extra costs but there may be several financial considerations and strains such as:

- giving up work or going part-time
- moving the bed downstairs or buying a new bed
- buying a suitable chair (a padded garden chair or recliner might be suitable in the short term)
- moving to more suitable housing
- extra heating bills
- transport costs – e.g. taxis if you don't drive
- private care to give you a break

You might be able to claim financial help. *See* 'Explore'.

Ask

The social worker will be able to advise you about benefits and welfare payments. Some are means tested, others are not and the regulations are subject to change. This is an area where the expertise of the social worker is invaluable and you should ask for their advice.

If travelling to hospital is causing financial strain, family members who are on Income Support, or have a very low income, may be eligible to apply to the Department of Work and Pensions for reimbursement of travel expenses. Even if they have a higher income, the social worker may be able to arrange for help.

Some hospitals and hospices have a volunteer coordinator, through whom you can contact a volunteer driver.

Occupational pension schemes

It is also worth asking the patient's employer about whether the patient's occupational pension scheme entitles them to any of the following:

- a pension before retirement age if they leave work due to illness
- death-in-service lump sum payments and a pension for the spouse or dependent children
- immediate lump sum payment if there are no dependents and the patient is terminally ill (the future pension is paid now in a lump sum which could pay for private care).

Note

Keep a note of the names and contact details of all the people who advise you about financial matters. It's easiest to talk to the same person if you need to update information or make a new claim if circumstances change.

Keep a note of the dates when the patient went off sick and any change in employment – e.g. temporary or permanent retirement. These details are sometimes asked for and are very hard to recall!

Do ✓

Keep photocopies of all important documents and any claim forms you or the patient fill in. This is the only way you can have an accurate record of what information you gave if there is a query at a later date when circumstances may have changed.

Explore

Sometimes there are other benefits and grants available. Here are some worth considering. This information can change, so check the details with the social worker.

Benefits payable to the patient

Attendance Allowance

This is a tax-free benefit for people aged 65 and over who require help with personal care due to illness or disability (*see* 'Disability Living Allowance'). It is payable at two levels, depending on the patient's needs. Normally to be eligible, the patient must have needed help with personal care for six months, but a claim may be made under 'special rules' if the patient is thought to have a short life expectancy. You, the carer, can apply on behalf of the patient if they are terminally ill. If the patient is unaware of their diagnosis, an application can still be made by the carer without the patient being told their prognosis.

Benevolent societies

There are various benevolent societies, particularly for ex-servicemen, retired actors and actresses and other groups. One of these may provide financial support for a suitable patient. Some societies will help with funeral costs and ex-service persons who are in receipt of a war pension may be able to claim help with the cost of a simple funeral if they died from the condition for which the pension was being paid. Further details may be obtained from The War Pensions Agency, Norcross, Blackpool FY5 3WP.

You might wish to contact the Soldiers, Sailors & Airmen Family Association, 19 Queen Elizabeth Street, London SE1 2LP.

Disability Living Allowance

It is advisable to consult a social worker to check for recent changes and amendments to welfare benefits, as these change fairly frequently.

Disability Living Allowance (care component) or Attendance Allowance for patients who are terminally ill is obtained under so-called 'special rules' using Form DS1500. A claim under 'special rules' can be made on behalf of a terminally ill patient even if they are unaware of the terminal nature of their condition – although it is usually better to discuss this with the patient prior to making the application.

Special provision is made within the Disability Living Allowance, for those under the age of 65, and with the Attendance Allowance, for those over 65, with a terminal illness. In order to do this, Form DS1500 is required which can be completed by the GP or hospital doctor. It can be obtained from the GP or the Macmillan nurse.

Macmillan Cancer Relief

You might like to contact the Macmillan Cancer Relief Information Line on 0845 601 6161. From Monday to Friday, 09.30–19.30, callers may obtain information about how to gain access to Macmillan services and how to contact other cancer-related organisations and support agencies.

If the patient has financial difficulties Macmillan grants may be made for any reasonable and practical necessity e.g.:

- clothing and footwear
- furnishings such as beds and suitable chairs
- essential equipment like a cooker, fridge, microwave or washing machine
- heating costs and short-term costs of care
- the cost of telephone installation or even overdue rent or mortgage payments.

Application forms are available from GPs, Macmillan palliative care nurses, social workers and district nurses.

Statutory Sick Pay (SSP)

SSP is paid by the employer for 28 weeks if the patient is unable to work due to illness or disability.

Incapacity Benefit

Incapacity Benefit is paid to people who cannot work due to illness or disability. The amount paid depends on National Insurance contributions and it normally stops when the patient reaches pensionable age.

Severe Disablement Allowance

This is paid to people who cannot get Incapacity Benefit because they have not paid enough National Insurance contributions.

Benefits payable to the carer

Invalid Care Allowance (ICA)

This benefit is payable to people aged between 16 and 65 if they cannot work because they are looking after someone at least 35 hours a week. To be eligible for ICA, your patient must be receiving Disability Living Allowance or Attendance Allowance. ICA 'overlaps' with other State benefits, so if you are already in receipt of these the amount of ICA payable may be reduced.

The Carer Premium

This is payable to someone already in receipt of Income Support, Housing Benefit or Council Tax Benefit. If you are entitled to ICA you can also claim Carer Premium.

More Information

Serious or prolonged illness is a financial strain. The State benefits may be less than you expected. If you are on a low income, it might be worth asking about

- Council Tax Benefit
- Housing Benefit
- Income Support
- NHS costs and how you may be exempt from certain charges
- prescription costs (a diagnosis of cancer does not qualify the patient for free prescriptions, but a continuing physical disability does [terminal illness can count] and it is worth obtaining form FP91 from the post office)
- the Social Fund.

The Citizens Advice Bureau or the social worker can offer up-to-date information.

If you, the carer, are working, think about how you would cope financially if you were to become a patient yourself. You might wish to think about some form of private insurance to cover illness, redundancy or loss of job. Hopefully you'll never need it, but it is a tax-exempt income that could be much needed if you were unfortunate enough to become seriously ill.

Plain Speaking: Communication

Chapter 7

The patient has been given bad news

The doctor says

You may be invited to be present at the appointment when the patient is given bad news. If so, it is likely that, in the discussion you will have with the patient afterwards, you will recall details that they did not pick up and they will talk about issues that you don't remember being mentioned. This is normal.

One criticism that has been made is that we doctors try to tell our patients too much at one appointment. I know that my mind went quite blank after I heard the word 'cancer'. I was already pretty sure I had cancer, but having someone else tell you is quite different. Then it is really true! What was just a fear is now reality. It's time to re-think your whole life – whether you are the patient or the carer – your future has changed.

It's very hard to take the whole message on board at one appointment. Having a second person present definitely helps, but it is still difficult to take in what is actually being said. The message is often life-changing.

It's very important to hear and understand what was said and what it meant. Background noise, the strange environment, awareness of pressure of time and talking to a complete stranger do not help. If you have any problem with your hearing or with understanding what is being said, say so! A hearing problem is nothing to be ashamed of. Too many patients smile, nod and give the impression that all is well but, in reality, they heard very little of what had been said. Nobody benefits – least of all, you and the patient.

Patients react in several different ways when they have been given bad news. Here are a few of the common reactions.

- **anger**: at life, God, oneself (e.g. blaming oneself for one's lifestyle)
- **despair**: no future: no hope of cure
- **disbelief**: it's all a big mistake
- **fear**: of the disease, treatment, suffering, death, etc.
- **gratitude**: for an honest discussion
- **optimism**: sometimes can be used as a defence mechanism
- **relief**: at last we know what exactly is wrong.

After a few days most patients begin to accept the reality of their diagnosis and begin to accept the facts. Sadness is common in the early stages; depression (Chapter 18) is less common than one would expect.

Think

While you will probably want to know as much as possible about the disease, the treatment and the likely outcome, I must remind you that the patient has the final say in how much you are told. The professional carers will only be able to discuss the patient's situation with their consent. To offer the best care you do need to know a certain amount and you need to think about these questions.

How much do you already know?

The important question here is what do you *know*: not what do you *think*. Is there something that you *think* might be wrong, but nobody has told you whether you are right or wrong? Ask the patient and, if necessary, seek their permission for a discussion with the doctor or nurse to enable you to offer the best care.

Who gave you that information?

If you do know something (in other words, you don't just think it), who told you the facts? Do you need to confirm any of the details?

If a doctor uses a word you don't understand, ask for an explanation. Equally, patients sometimes use medical terms that they have picked up during their hospital visits throughout their illness. Make sure that you understand what the patient means. Your understanding of the term may be different. One of you might even have misunderstood it. Nobody benefits in such circumstances. Don't assume – ask.

Does the patient want you to be present to make sure they heard everything and that they heard it correctly?

It certainly can help, but you can't force the patient to agree to your presence.

The first time I was told 'bad news' I had left my wife, Alice, in the waiting room. Alice accompanies me on all significant interviews now. She has heard things that I didn't hear because I had 'switched off'. In our discussion afterwards, we both get 'the whole message'. Likewise, I have attended many appointments with her and I sometimes recalled bits of information that she had missed.

The doctor may ask the patient if they are happy for you to be present. This is not because they object to your presence in any way but simply because they are obliged, under laws of medical confidentiality, to check. Your presence probably indicates that the patient is happy for you to hear what is discussed, but since the information is confidential between the patient and the doctor, they may decide to confirm that that patient is happy for you to be present.

If requested, a nurse can also be present and she can help you afterwards with any issues that you need to re-check or clarify.

Ask

If you went with the patient when they were given bad news, there are probably many questions you want to ask. You need to be aware that the news was given to the patient and they need to have the opportunity to ask the questions they want answered. The doctor may be less enthusiastic about allowing you to be 'spokesperson'.

It might be appropriate to have a discussion with the patient after the interview and then arrange to speak to the family doctor or a specialist nurse to clarify areas where you need more information.

Always be aware that you might wish to ask about issues that the patient is not ready or willing to discuss. The staff are obliged to respect their wishes in this regard.

Note

Encourage the patient to make a note of anything that you both need to ask about. You might wish to enquire about the kind of care the patient will need during treatment or if the disease progresses.

Do ✔

You might find it helpful to bring a pen and some paper with you. A few key words can act as a memory-jogger later.

Explore

It is quite likely that, a couple of days after your first appointment, you and the patient will have questions that you want answered. Recognising that it takes a few days for letters to be typed and sent back to your family doctor, you might wish to explore these issues.

- Do you need to make another appointment to discuss anything – e.g. results of tests?
- Who else could offer advice? Is there a specialist nurse that could help? Will they have access to the patient's notes and the relevant details?

As you sit at home over the next day or two, you will be thinking about the news you have been given. You will probably be asking yourself the following questions:

- Have you been given all the information you want or need (assuming it is currently available)?
- Did you understand what was said?
- Did you ask about who is available to offer support and clarify what you discussed?

If the answer to any of these is 'no', make a note of the things you need to ask at your next appointment.

More Information

Giving a patient bad news is one of the hardest things a doctor has to do. The doctor's aim in this 'bad news' appointment is to:

- explore what the patient knows about their illness
- discuss treatment plans
- answer questions about the illness, the treatment and the longer-term outlook. Remember, things can change.

In the early stages, your exact role as a carer may be hard to define and, initially, support may be the main need. As the patient becomes weak and tired as a result of the treatment, your role will change. It may not be possible to predict the patient's needs at this early stage.

Chapter 8

You know the patient has cancer before they do

The doctor says

It is usual for the patient to be the first to be told they have cancer, but occasionally the situation arises where the family knows first. Professional carers know the results of tests before the patient does, but they don't usually tell the relatives first. Relatives have asked me to 'tell us, but don't tell the patient'. What should one do in this situation?

As a general rule, the patient should be told their diagnosis and the treatment options. It is up to them to decide who else is told and what they are told. Some patients share all the information, some say little or nothing. It is not up to the staff to share information with a 'third party' without the patient's consent.

Professional carers will often be aware of results of tests before the patient is. Results are delivered to clinics and wards and in the course of being filed in the patient's notes, they may be seen by clerical and clinical staff. Staff working in these areas are expected to respect the confidentiality of information and not 'jump the gun' by speaking to the patient or relatives before they are seen by the relevant clinician, but obviously 'leaks' of information do occur.

Assuming that the patient is of mature years and of sound mind, what do you do if you hear the diagnosis first?

Think

Who told you or how did you find out?

It's not easy giving someone 'bad news', so it's probably best for you to wait until the doctor tells the patient, but it is difficult not to let something show that you know. There may have been a breach of the usual rules of confidentiality, but would the patient wish to pursue this? You could be in trouble for asking or colluding with the person who told you.

Can you get the patient's treatment started any faster by knowing these results?

Generally speaking, even when you know the results of tests, you can't speed up the process of starting treatment. There are other patients who are just as sick who are also waiting to start their treatment. An expert who will see the results will decide the most appropriate course of action. It's natural to worry because you know something needs to be done, but this simply adds to your natural anxiety while achieving nothing useful.

As a doctor, I received no priority over others on waiting lists – they were just as sick as I was and I believe it was right for me to treated as the consultant saw appropriate to my needs and theirs.

Ask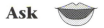

If someone wishes to give you the diagnosis before telling the patient, ask yourself (and them) why they are doing this.

What is the advantage, to the patient and to you, for you to be the first to know?

Note

Make a note of exactly what you were told, who said it and when. The patient may ask you for these details later on.

Do ✓

Try to avoid being told about the patient before the patient is told their own diagnosis. Exceptions to this rule are children for whom you have to make decisions and those who cannot make decisions for themselves, possibly due to a learning disability.

My personal advice is that you make every attempt to ensure that the patient is told first (unless they are not competent to be told). Every attempt should made to respect the patient's right to be told about their illness first and then to decide who else needs to be told and how much they need to know. Patients can lose trust in their professional carers if they believe their personal details are being discussed with 'third parties'. Don't fall into the trap. Nobody benefits and it simply causes problems.

Explore

Are any issues that you need to explore before the patient is told their diagnosis, e.g. where they can be cared for if you cannot accept this responsibility at this time? This might be the time to do so if it ensures that the patient will be less anxious when they do get to hear their diagnosis and the treatment plan.

More Information

If the patient is less than about 16 years old you'll probably be told first or you and the child might be told together.

If the patient is suffering from a learning disability or other illness that affects their ability to understand the implications of the diagnosis, you might be told first or at the same time as the patient.

In both of these cases, you will probably be used to taking responsibility for and making decisions on behalf of the patient.

Elderly patients who are mentally competent are usually told their diagnosis and old age alone is not a reason for relatives and carers to be told first or exclusively. My experience is that some people seem to think that old people can't handle bad news, but I disagree and feel that they need to be aware of the truth so they can deal with personal business in the remaining time they have.

Chapter 9

The staff don't seem to have time to speak to me

This chapter is basically about patients in hospital, but the same principles apply to patients at home with various professionals visiting and offering care.

The doctor says

Recently, when visiting my wife in hospital, I was very aware of the numbers of nurses and doctors rushing about. Which ones were dealing with Alice? Who should I speak to? Who knows most about her?

It is not easy for staff to answer questions about a patient they do not know and I have known relatives who thought the staff were purposely avoiding them. Let me say from experience that even the very best notes are not a substitute for knowing the patient personally.

Thankfully, on this occasion, the consultant appeared and my problem was resolved. We had a three-person discussion at the bedside.

When my wife was ill, the doctor would not speak to me until she had obtained Alice's permission. This is done to protect the patient's confidentiality and right to privacy.

Telephone enquiries present a particular problem because of the problems of being able to identify the caller and often staff will be very reluctant to discuss anything by phone.

Think

You might wish to speak to a staff member for the first time or as a follow-up to previous discussions. In either case, it might be worth considering these basic questions first.

What do you need to discuss?

Spend a few minutes thinking about what you need to ask about or discuss with the doctor or nurse. It might help you to make a note of the things you need to talk about. This makes you more focused and reduces the risk of forgetting something.

When do you need to know?

Is it essential for you to have the information immediately, or could you wait a day or two? Sometimes we need time to plan, arrange and make necessary changes and we need information immediately. There are other times when we could wait a day or two to see the member of staff who is best able to advise us. Think about whether you can afford to wait to see the person most able to advise you.

Who else could give you this information?

If the situation is such that you need information now, ask who else can advise you. Occasionally you might be given information to 'get you started' and be asked to arrange a second meeting to find out about specific details.

Why do you need to see the doctor or nurse?

Is it to find out something new, or to clarify something that you discussed previously? Perhaps someone else could answer the question if it is something you have not discussed previously. If it is a follow-up on a previous discussion, ask when is a convenient time to meet the doctor or nurse you spoke to previously.

Ask

If you cannot see the person you wish to see now, ask about:

- returning at a mutually agreeable time
- whether another member of the team could help.

If you need to ask something urgently, ask whether you could have a very brief chat now and possibly book a longer appointment later.

   If the person you wish to speak to seems to be reluctant to see you, ask whether the patient has refused to give their permission for you to speak to the staff. If this is the case, speak to the patient about why you want to speak to the staff, what it is you want to know and how it will help you to care for them. It is their right to refuse to allow you to speak to the staff. Some patients are happy for relatives to have information relevant to their practical needs and care, but not about the illness and how they are responding to treatment.

Note

Make a note of the information you need and questions you want to ask.

   It is probably best to agree with the patient about the issues that you want to ask about and, if necessary, why you need to know.

   Make a note of the person to whom you spoke and the date of your discussion. Things can change very quickly and sometimes it is easy to think we misunderstood the message. If there is any question over what was said, knowing who spoke to you can help in clarifying any issues that seem to have changed since that conversation.

Do ☑

- Respect the patient's right to privacy.
- Recognise that you might have to wait a short time to see the member of staff who knows the patient best and can give you the best information and advice.
- Remember that it might be best to make an appointment for the discussion to allow adequate time and a private place to talk.

- Allow the patient to be present. Your request to see a doctor or nurse alone may be refused. *See* Chapter 11 'Avoiding collusion with the patient'.

Explore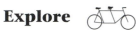

- Is someone else available who could speak to you?
- Is it possible to arrange to visit the patient when the doctor or nurse will be available?
- If things are changing and you feel the need to have regular discussions, is it possible to agree a pattern of mutually acceptable times for such updates?

More Information

It is not uncommon for people to think that staff do not wish to speak to them. One must remember that the staff can't usually 'make the first move'. If the staff are reluctant to enter into discussion it is probably because the patient has not given specific consent or they simply have nothing new to tell you.

Chapter 10

There is not enough privacy for discussions with the staff

The doctor says

The patient's bedside is not a particularly private place. Older hospitals often had little opportunity for privacy except for a curtain round the bed. Most hospitals now do have a room somewhere where one can have a quiet confidential conversation. It always pays to ask, especially if either you or the patient have any difficulty in hearing. Hospital wards are also busy noisy places and you probably would find it much easier to be less distracted by the goings on around you.

Think

- What do you want to talk about? This helps you decide how much privacy is needed.
- How much time do you think you will need? You might need to book the room in advance and should allow yourself adequate time. It might involve waiting a little longer for a room and the appropriate staff member to be available, but should be worth the effort.
- Will you be discussing any kind of 'bad news' or something that might be emotionally difficult for you or the patient? If so, it may be worth exploring the availability of a private room and some time afterwards for you to spend some time alone together, away from the other patients.

Ask

- Are there any physical problems, e.g. deafness, that could compromise one's privacy at the bedside? If so, ask the staff for an appropriate room where you can talk without being overheard.
- If the patient is in bed, can they be brought to a room in a wheelchair or even their bed? If not, what else can be done to ensure adequate privacy?

Note

Before the discussion, make a note of all the things you wish to discuss. Make sure that the patient is happy for these to be discussed – they have the right to refuse and the staff must respect the wishes of a competent patient.

Do

Find out if the patient would like their named nurse or another person to be present with them. You might raise something that they have not thought about and they might wish to discuss it again later. Patients can be easily tired and can't always retain everything that is said, so do be prepared for an advocate to be present. Their presence does not undermine your role: they can be present when you are not and they may have access to essential information that the patient needs.

Explore

The main things to explore are:

- What is to be discussed? The patient must agree with this 'agenda'.
- Who should be present at the discussion? The patient must agree with this.
- Where should discussions take place to ensure privacy acceptable to the patient and you?
- When can the discussion take place?

You might be responsible for setting up the discussion, but always with the patient's consent.

More Information

It is always possible that, during a discussion where several people are present, something will be mentioned that was not previously known to someone. This should not become a reason for undue anxiety – it's easy for the patient to forget to mention something or even not hear it in the first place.

The staff will also be very careful to avoid any form of collusion or requests 'not to tell the patient' (*see* Chapter 11). All the issues discussed are about the patient and the competent patient has the right to know what is going on and to decide who else should be involved in their illness.

Avoiding collusion with the patient

The doctor says

Collusion, in this context, usually refers to a request from a relative for members of staff not to tell the patient his or her diagnosis and the likely outcome of treatment. While people who make such requests do not set out to cause any trouble and have only the best intentions in mind, such actions cause many problems.

Requests of this type are usually made with the intention of protecting the patient from being upset by hearing bad news. Far from protecting the patient, collusion usually generates secondary communication problems.

The staff must respect the competent patient's autonomy and respect their right to be told what is wrong with them.

Think

If someone, including yourself, thinks that the patient should not be made aware of their diagnosis and the possible outcomes of treatment etc., think about the following issues. The length of this section indicates how carefully one needs to think before deciding to enter into any form of collusion.

Why should the patient not be told?

- Is it because you think they will not understand the message? Someone with a severe learning disability might fit into this category, but old age is not always a reason to withhold information. Confusion can improve and elderly people sometimes have lucid periods between times of being forgetful or a bit confused.

  If it is decided that the patient is not fit to understand the diagnosis and treatment options, this decision should be made by more than one close family member and agreed with the senior staff responsible for the patient's care. A detailed record of the discussion should be recorded in the patient's notes and there are clear implications concerning future decisions about care, finances, a will, etc.
- Do you believe that the patient would not cope with the bad news or are you afraid of causing them undue distress?
- Are you having difficulty in accepting the truth and coming to terms with the news yourself? Are you afraid to have an open discussion with the patient?
- Do you, or any of the family, or the patient hope that if you deny the problem, it could perhaps go away? It won't!

Failure to communicate may cause isolation, both of the patient and of the family, with everyone scared to be open and honest with the other.

How has the patient coped with difficult situations in the past?

How people coped in the past can be a useful indicator of how they will cope with a new problem. If they didn't cope well, it might be tempting to 'protect' them from the truth. On the other hand, a serious illness requiring planning for the future may be something that they want to deal with themselves and it may be impossible for you to judge this without a frank discussion.

Think about these questions:

- What do you and the patient's relatives think will happen if the patient is made aware of his or her disease?
- Would the patient wish family members to be aware of his or her disease and prognosis and be available to help with any personal business?
- What is the current relationship between the patient, you and other family members?
- How are other members of the family coping with this situation, and how do they think this current situation should be handled?

Who should decide that the patient is not told?

Usually such requests come from close family members. It is usually assumed that the patient is unaware of their diagnosis, but experience shows that this is often not the case and the patient often has already suspected what is wrong.

It is possible for a 'cycle of protection' to become established in which the patient seeks to protect the family from the truth and the family seeks to protect the patient. This invariably leads to problems for the patient, who may be unable to 'let go' or talk about feelings. The surviving family members may experience difficulties in bereavement, having not said 'goodbye' to their loved one and being left with unfinished business to resolve.

Think very carefully about who will be left with this responsibility and the feelings of guilt and blame that may be associated with the decision 'not to tell'.

What should the patient be told?

Patients can often guess their diagnosis and, while they really need their suspicions to be confirmed or refuted, they might be reluctant to ask.

As a medical student, I was taught three basic 'ground rules' about what to tell patients about their diagnosis and the likely outcome of their illness.

- You will always tell the truth if asked.
- You will not tell if the patient tells you that he or she does not want to hear, and you can only tell the relatives if the patient agrees.
- You will always have the patient as your primary concern and will respect their wishes before agreeing to requests from relatives.

It is important to realise some basic facts.

- Sometimes the patient's fears and anxieties can be worse than the actual diagnosis. (I've 'been there' and speak from experience!)
- Sometimes, unfounded fears and anxieties can be dealt with effectively by knowing the truth.
- You and the other relatives are probably communicating non-verbally already! Our eye contact (or lack of it) and general body language can 'give the game away'. Our body language is often more honest than our speech!
- At any stage of the illness, the patient relates to various people as well as their family. The professional carers will wish to avoid misunderstandings and will not want to be involved in collusion. How do you know that someone else has not told the patient the truth?
- Undoubtedly your motive will be based on love and protecting the patient, but collusion can cause a barrier. Creating barriers, especially during the final part of life, can result in increased bereavement problems and extra 'unfinished business' to deal with after a death.

When should the patient be told the truth?

If, after all this thinking, you decide that the patient should not be told the truth yet, when should they be told and by whom?

If family members have asked for the truth to be withheld initially, staff may not wish to take on the role of breaking the bad news later on. Since they were not the ones who wanted to withhold the information, why should they be given this task now?

A few more things to think about.

- How do you decide what is a good time to tell the truth? Do you wait until it is obvious that the patient will not get better and thus waste time in which they could have achieved some desired goal that is not possible now? Do you wait until they start some kind of treatment that one associates with cancer?
- Withholding information as a 'protection mechanism' can cause problems when one decides, at some point, to admit that information had been withheld. Time has been lost during which the patient could have been thinking about putting their affairs in order, making their peace with God and preparing for their death.
- The family may have been suppressing their own grief to present a controlled front. This causes enormous stress and potential problems within families.
- How do you know that the patient was not fully aware of the diagnosis but trying to protect you by remaining silent?

Ask

If you now believe that the patient should know the diagnosis, you need not be alone in helping them cope with the news. There are people you can ask for help: for instance, members of staff with whom the patient has a good rapport. Talk with them to discuss the situation with them and share your concerns about how the patient might react to their diagnosis.

Acknowledge the patient's right for you not to be told the outcome of any discussion they have with the staff. This is not easy, but it does allow better communication between the patient and the doctor or nurse. You must trust them to do their job well and offer appropriate support, even if you are not involved as much as you'd like to be.

Note

If it has been agreed that information will not be withheld, but will be given to the patient slowly to allow them time to come to terms with it, make sure that you keep a note of what they have been told and make sure that other family members are aware of this too. In such cases you want to make sure that you and the staff work together to ensure that:

- staff and relatives will take cues from the patient on the amount and nature of information given and the pace with which it is given
- information will not be given without proper support being made available
- relatives and staff will tell the patient the truth should he or she ask what is happening to them.

Do ✔

- Continue to visit and provide support for the patient and other family members. It is not easy to cope with a situation where one is coming to terms with a serious illness and everyone needs support, whether they agree with the current course of action or not.
- Discuss the care arrangements with different professionals e.g. doctors, nurses and social workers to make sure that you know what is going on.
- Avoid conflicting opinions with the patient if possible.

Explore

If some family members still insist that the patient should not be told their diagnosis, you should explore the following issues.

- What is their reason for suggesting this course of action?
- What effect will this action have on the patient?
- What effect will this action have on other relatives?
- What effect will this action have on present and future family interaction?
- What are the rights and needs of the patient?

Accurate information is the right of the patient – it is his or her disease. The patient has the right both to have the information and to withhold it from others.

More Information

Collusion is probably the most common problem in early stages of disease and shortly after diagnosis. At this stage, one common coping mechanism is to deny the reality of the problem. This is not a reason for keeping the truth from the patient. Sometimes it becomes the basis for colluding on a short-term basis while the truth 'sinks in'.

If families insist on or persist in colluding, it may be the role of the professionals to intervene and sensitively dismantle the collusion. By practising honesty and encouraging both patient and family in their expression of feelings, the staff will try to encourage and facilitate more open communication for all. On the other hand, the staff are not there to 'rescue' family members who become embroiled in avoidable conflict.

You can only support the patient and family members effectively if there is a good dialogue between the patient, the staff and all the family members, while recognising and respecting the rights of the patient in their freedom of choice and their right to privacy.

Section 3

Practical Problems

Chapter 12

The patient has a very poor appetite

The doctor says

Almost any serious illness and many forms of treatment, including chemotherapy or radiotherapy for cancer, can cause loss of appetite. Following chemotherapy, taste may be altered, appetite reduced and one can develop an aversion to some foods or tea and coffee. This generally improves with time but one cannot predict how long it will persist.

Chewing one's food can be very exhausting and sometimes a soft diet is better tolerated in the period following treatment.

Sometimes this loss of appetite causes more distress to the patient's relatives than the patient themselves. There is a tendency for us to want to 'build the patient up' and to encourage eating more. Often smaller meals with simple snacks in between are better.

Think

What is causing the loss of appetite? Make a note of any of the following points that apply:

- altered taste (can occur with some chemotherapy and after radiotherapy to the head and neck)
- constipation
- dislike of the food offered (too rich/too spicy/too bland, etc.)
- exhaustion
- fear of being sick or an 'upset tummy'
- meals offered are too big and this gives the *impression* of a poor appetite
- mouth problems – sore, dry or oral thrush infection
- nausea and vomiting
- radiotherapy to the abdomen
- swallowing problems
- treatment known to cause loss of appetite e.g. chemotherapy.

Ask

Ask about any of the issues identified in the 'Think' section, but also ask about the following:

- What is the patient's normal appetite? Too big a meal can be very off-putting and can make one suddenly not feel hungry!

- What does the patient want to eat? Sometimes one develops food cravings. Other times one wants something simple and easy to eat which may not be what was 'planned' by the relative or carer.
- Does the patient have a preferred pattern for eating – big breakfast, small evening meal, or vice versa?
- Is there a time of day when the patient's appetite is better than another time of day?

Note

Make a note of food likes and dislikes and the times of day when the appetite is best. Try to make use of food preferences to offer a suitable choice of meal at a time when the patient is most likely to enjoy it.

If a particular brand of a food is better tolerated or tastes better to the patient, make a note of this. Tastes can alter during treatment and revert to 'normal' later.

Do

- Explore, with the patient, what foods they like best.
- Try foods that are bland if the patient's mouth is sore.
- Offer a small aperitif, e.g. sherry (if alcohol is allowed).
- Offer small appetising meals, on a smaller plate.
- Offer soft moist food if the patient's mouth is dry or there is any difficulty in swallowing.
- Offer a fizzy drink with the meal if the patient has had a tube inserted in the oesophagus (gullet) to overcome an obstruction.
- Try not to expose the patient to cooking smells, which can be responsible for loss of appetite or nausea. When cooking cabbage or sprouts, a small bay leaf added to the water greatly reduces the cooking smell and the smell of cauliflower cooking is reduced by adding lemon to the saucepan (traditionally half of the 'shell' of a squeezed lemon). You'll find some more tips about cooking smells in Chapter 31.

When eating out

- Try children's portions if eating out. (I have never had any problem ordering a child's meal when I explained the reason for doing so.)
- Ask for extra sauce, mayonnaise or butter if a meal is a bit dry.

Explore

Try to find ways of adding extra calories to food without adding to the amount the patient can eat. You'll find a few ideas to get you started below in the section 'Some ways to add extra calories and protein to your meals'.

More Information 📖

Trying to encourage a patient to eat more when it's the thing they least feel like doing can be a cause of stress to both patient and carer. You'll find some tried and tested ideas on the next few pages.

Sometimes, when patients cannot swallow, possibly due to a tumour blocking the gullet, a tube is inserted into the stomach. These 'percutaneous endoscopic gastrostomy' (PEG) tubes allow special food supplements to be delivered directly into the stomach. The tube is placed in position under anaesthetic and, after an initial period to allow everything to settle, can remain there for a long time.

If it can be arranged for the patient to have their 'feed' at night, one can be free to move around and even go out during the day. The dietician will advise about the most suitable food supplement for the individual patient.

Some ways to add extra calories and protein to meals

- **Butter** can be added to cooked rice, cooked pasta and vegetables, etc. This adds some calories, fats and vitamins.
- **Buttering** toast while it's hot allows it to absorb more butter and therefore the patient gets more calories, fats and vitamins.
- **Creamers** (the type usually added to coffee) add calcium, glucose and vegetable fat.
- **Dried milk** added to ordinary milk (one cup per pint) doubles the protein content.
- **Mayonnaise** is fattier and has more calories than salad dressing.
- **Milk** can be used instead of water to dilute 'condensed' soups.
- **Soured cream** or cheese on potatoes adds extra calories and fats.
- **Sugar** can be added to cereals, or syrup to porridge, as a source of extra energy.
- **Vitamin drops** or medicines (the type usually bought for babies and very young children) may be used to provide extra vitamins. They can be added to food. Remember always to check the label and use exactly the amount recommended. Use a child's dose if you aren't sure. Cooking or heating destroys many vitamins, so the drops are best added after cooking or else added to foods not needing to be cooked.
- **Whipped cream** is full of calories and is easy to swallow. Add it to desserts and puddings.

Tips for improving the patient's appetite

- **An aperitif**, in the form of a small alcoholic drink, may help. If the patient is on medication, check that it is OK for them to have alcohol. Sometimes alcohol can interfere with the action of the medicine. Some cancer patients become intolerant of alcohol and may even experience pain after having a drink. 'Everything in moderation' is a good maxim. If the patient feels unwell or experiences pain after drinking even a small amount of alcohol, my personal advice is to advise them to do without the drink!

- **Cravings** for certain foods are fascinating and irritating. When I experienced food cravings, I initially tried to resist, but gradually I gave in and began to see that my body was probably in need of certain basic minerals or ingredients in those foods. As I began to recover, the cravings subsided. Some of the cravings never returned.

  My food cravings ranged from fried eggs to battered fish, fresh vegetable soup (every day for about four months) and fresh garden peas! Peas at breakfast time sounds a bit odd and I have no idea what my body lacked, but I don't really care because I felt better after the peas or fish and after a few days the cravings went away. Interestingly, when having chemotherapy, both Alice and I craved savoury and fatty foods like pies and pasties.

- **Encourage** the patient to eat when they are hungry. Their appetite might not be in rhythm with the family's normal mealtimes, but for a short spell, it might be possible to re-arrange the family routine or let the patient eat when their body tells them to. Their appetite may be best in the morning and decrease as the day progresses. Encourage them to 'listen to what their body says' and not to worry about family routines.

- **Exercising** before meals, if they are fit, will stimulate the patient's appetite. Fresh air is an added benefit. Even a few minutes spent sitting in the fresh air can help and may be worth the effort if they feel up to it. It also helps avoid the smell of food cooking, which can have a negative effect on appetite.

- **Fruit juice** or lemonade stimulates the appetite. If the patient has a sore mouth, these might make it even more painful. If this happens, avoid all fizzy drinks. Remember, even sugar-free fizzy drinks damage their teeth!

- **Individual food preferences**: having company and where you eat can all enhance the desire to eat or drink. Encourage the patient to eat the things they like and enjoy. If necessary, you can add a few more calories and protein by using the tips on the previous page. If they like to eat with others and enjoy company at mealtimes, try and arrange this, even for one meal each day.

- **Keep food out of sight** in between mealtimes. The sight of food can make patients feel sick. If their appetite is poor, the sight of food can act as a constant reminder of this problem and can make them feel much worse.

- **Small portions**, attractively served, are more appetising. If eating out, most restaurants will happily serve small portions on request. Many will also omit or add a particular food on request.

- **Snacks**, to nibble when desired, help improve one's food intake. Grated cheese, crisps, dried fruit and nuts or yoghurt are good choices.

Altered taste and loss of appetite

Chemotherapy and radiotherapy can affect how foods taste. Women who are suffering from cancer might notice that they experience the same changes in appetite and taste that they did during pregnancy.

Sometimes, simple ideas can help. The following tips might look and sound a bit odd, but be assured, they have all been used successfully.

- **Planning ahead**: during treatment patients are too tired to be bothered with cooking. If they cook for themselves, encourage them to plan ahead before starting a particularly tiring session of treatments. Sizeable quantities of dishes can be prepared that can be easily thawed and heated. If these are made in one-meal sized portions, they can be used when they feel unable to cope with cooking. Make some meals a bit smaller than their usual portion in case their appetite is affected. Alternatively, a stock of 'convenience foods' and frozen meals may save them some time and effort in preparation.
- **Cold food** has less taste than warm food and is worth trying.
- **Herbal teas** can be acceptable and pleasant, taken hot or cold.
- **Mints and boiled sweets** may give an acceptable taste in the mouth. Be aware of the increased risk of dental decay and the fact that hard sweets can cut and ulcerate their tongue and mouth, especially if their mouth is dry.
- **New flavours** are worth a try. The patient's tastes might have changed. Sometimes bland foods become better tolerated, especially during treatment. Radiotherapy affecting the head and neck can cause a sore mouth and sometimes very bland food is easiest to eat. Some types of chemotherapy can also cause a sore mouth and strong flavours and spicy foods can sting. These can appear to affect the 'appetite' because avoidance of food means less discomfort!
- **Plastic utensils** are not only for picnics and fast food outlets! Some chemotherapy drugs can give patients a metallic taste in the mouth. Using a normal metal fork or spoon can make this seem worse, but using plastic utensils may reduce this unpleasant sensation and allow the patient to enjoy their food better.
- **Sauces and marinades** can add moistness and flavour, both of which are lost if one has a dry mouth. Choose bland flavours if the patient's mouth is sore.
- **Spices** can be added to disguise tastes that are not being tolerated too well, but patients are often more than usually sensitive to spicy foods.

Chapter 13

The patient is breathless

The doctor says

Feeling short of breath is probably one of the most frightening problems one can experience. Sufferers feel frightened and anxious and we, the carers, feel powerless to help.

There are some practical things we can do to make life a bit easier for the patient, but one thing to clarify right at the outset is that inhalers (or 'puffers') are not usually the answer for cancer patients. Equally, oxygen is only helpful for a few carefully selected cancer sufferers and you must not feel that anyone is being neglectful because these have not been offered. They simply will not help.

Think

- How long has the patient been short of breath? If it is of recent onset or getting worse and the doctor has not been informed, suggest that the patient should see the doctor without delay.
- Do you (or the patient) know the cause of the shortness of breath and what can be done about it?
- Do you know whether the problem is expected to stay the same, get worse, or get better? If a change is expected, do you have an idea of what might happen?
- Do you know what to do if the patient's breathing worsens suddenly?

Ask

Does the patient get breathless

- Sitting resting?
- On lying flat?
- Only when trying to do something?

If the patient has a cough

- Did it start recently?
- Is he or she coughing up sputum (phlegm) and, if so, has this changed in volume or colour? Yellow or green sputum suggests a chest infection.
- Are they coughing up blood?

If the patient suffers from pain in their chest

- Is it there all the time?
- Do they only get chest pain when they try to take any form of exercise?
- Do they only get chest pain when they take a deep breath or cough?

If any of these have changed or are getting worse, check that the doctor or nurse has been informed.

Note

Make a note of any changes you see in the patient's breathing.

Compile a list of any questions you need to ask (with the patient's consent, of course).

Note any things that seem to help – e.g. a cooler room, a particular position or relaxing music or some other form of distraction.

Do

Agree with the patient how you can offer practical help. You might meet with some resistance, because one always fights to retain 'normality' by doing things for oneself.

- Place a chair at the bottom and top of the stairs or mid way between bathroom and bedroom to 'break the journey' if walking these distances makes the patient exhausted and short of breath.
- Offer to do any fetching and carrying for them. Carrying even relatively light items can be enough to make manageable shortness of breath intolerable.
- Help the patient find a comfortable position. Being propped up at about 45 degrees is often the best position.
- Adjust room temperatures to what suits the patient best (usually cooler rather than warmer).
- Try a fan blowing cool air near, but not directly at, the patient's face. Oscillating fans are best, if available.
- Encourage the patient to do things slowly and to rest as often as required.
- Help the patient to relax! It's easy to say, but very hard to do. Try soothing music and encourage them to breathe slowly and steadily.
- Encourage the patient to focus their attention on something else and not on their breathing.
- Slow down and go at the patient's pace when doing things together. Being left behind is stressful to patients and makes them aware of their difficulties. If they must do things like shopping, choose the least busy times and try to avoid the hustle and bustle of busy shops, which can make one feel worse. Alice and I found that shopping centres, with no fresh air, made us feel quite claustrophobic and we found it easier when the shops were less crowded and we were able to complete our shopping more quickly.
- If possible, anticipate the things that make the patient breathless and plan how to minimise the amount of effort they need to make to achieve the desired goal.

Explore

Simple comfort measures like a gentle hand and arm massage can help. Acupuncture can also help but may not be available on the NHS and could be quite expensive. Always choose qualified practitioners (*see* Appendix 4, 'Useful organisations') but don't forget that simple measures to improve comfort and reduce anxiety are very effective.

More Information

Getting comfortable in bed can be difficult and it is sometimes worth looking into the value of an adjustable bed which allows the patient to position themselves so that their breathing is easiest. Many people have found these beneficial, but before purchasing, why not ask for a trial, with a written guarantee of a full refund if it is not suitable?

If the patient has lung cancer, you might be wondering about their fitness to drive.

People who hold a LGV licence should ask their doctor or DVLA about their fitness to continue driving the LGV. They should report a diagnosis of lung cancer made within the past two years and may need to produce evidence of fitness to drive.

To check about notifiable medical conditions and see updated information from DVLA, look at their website www.dvla.gov.uk/drivers/dmed1.

Chapter 14

The patient is having chemotherapy

The doctor says

Chemotherapy is the use of medicines to kill cancer cells. The drugs may be given in tablet form but are often given as a drip into a vein and treatments can take anything from a few minutes to several hours to administer. Because the drugs must be freshly made up in a specially controlled environment, it can take a couple of hours to prepare the prescription. This means that the patient could wait an hour or so after seeing the doctor before starting their treatment session. Bring a good book, a drink and a snack if necessary!

It is common for the patient to be given tablets to take for a few days after the treatment session. These drugs usually include something for sickness, a steroid to reduce the reaction to treatment and sometimes other medications. Steroids, especially in higher doses, can cause restlessness and some degree of agitation. They can affect one's sleep, so to avoid sleep disruption it is best if the last dose is taken around 6pm. Steroids often stimulate the patient's appetite.

Think

Chemotherapy is usually given as an outpatient or a day patient, although patients occasionally stay in hospital, either overnight, or for a few days for a more complicated regime. Side effects such as sickness are usually worst in the days immediately following treatment and it is at these times that the patient might need extra support and care.

It might help you plan if you think about the following issues:

- How frequently is treatment being given?
- How many treatments are planned?
- Do you have the days and dates for the treatments?
- Can you be available for a few days after each of these sessions, should that prove necessary?
- Are there any important events in your personal diary that might affect your availability to offer care?

Ask

There are some practical issues that you might like to discuss to ensure you are ready to take on the practical care of the patient.

- What are the likely side effects of the treatment?
- How long will these last?

- What do you do if the medications given to control any side effects do not work: do you contact the GP or a hospital clinical specialist nurse for advice?
- If you have identified an event that prevents you from being available to offer care, and nobody else is available, can the treatment dates be adjusted to suit this without compromising the effects of the treatment? If not, what alternative arrangements can be made to make sure the patient is cared for?

Note

From the questions asked above, make a note of any issues you need to discuss further. If there is an aspect of the practical care that is likely to cause you particular difficulty or is something you do not feel able to do, make a note of this. Discuss it with the nurse or doctor so that appropriate arrangements are made for the proper care of the patient.

You must not feel guilty about anything you feel unable to do – you are not expected to be able to offer the same input as a professional carer.

Make a note of the side effects of treatment – e.g. nausea, constipation, etc. – when these started, how long they lasted and what helped to alleviate the symptoms. Ask the doctor or nurse about how to manage or prevent these problems as they will probably happen after each session of treatment.

Some people suffer food cravings during chemotherapy treatment. Make a note of these if they occur and be prepared for the next time! I wanted fresh garden peas for breakfast; my wife craved Chinese chicken and sweetcorn soup and rice pudding at 3am!

Do ☑

Be prepared for the patient to feel quite unwell for a few days after each dose of chemotherapy. They might need help because they are:

- Constipated: This often settles after a day or two, but if it is causing distress, speak to the nurse or doctor. Constipation can make nausea and vomiting worse.
- Emotionally upset: Poor sleep and feeling sick, weak and tired all contribute to a poor quality of life for a few days. The first pulse of chemotherapy is the one when one least knows what to expect, so after that one can roughly anticipate what will happen, but do remember that tiredness often gets worse as treatment progresses and one becomes anaemic and generally run down.
- Having food cravings: Women may find these similar to those they experienced during pregnancy. Many people find that their cravings need to be satisfied very quickly or they feel very agitated and anxious.
- Nauseated or vomiting: Keep a suitable receptacle handy. A 2 litre ice-cream container is useful for the car journey home and a supermarket carrier bag (without any holes) acts as a useful liner and makes cleaning up easier later. Some people find that sucking crystallized ginger helps car-sickness.
- Sleeping badly at night or needing to have a drink or snack during the night if they cannot eat normally during the day.

- Tired: Many patients need to rest for a while during the day. Set aside a time each day when you do not allow people to visit so that the patient has adequate rest and sleep. This can also be the opportunity for you to 'catch up'. If you decide to go to the shops, put a note on the door asking callers not to ring the bell but to come back later. Disconnect the phone for a couple of hours if necessary!
- Unable to drink very much without feeling sick: Try different drinks – sometimes isotonic 'sports drinks' are easily taken and better tolerated than tea or coffee.
- Unable to eat very much: Simple small meals can help. Sometimes small frequent snacks are best tolerated for the first few days. *See* Chapter 12 'The patient has a very poor appetite' for further ideas.
- Weak and unsteady: Be prepared to accompany them up and down stairs.

Many treatments are associated with some degree of increased susceptibility to infection. Advise visitors who have colds and infections to 'keep their distance' until they are fully recovered.

Explore

It might be appropriate for you to find out more about the treatment the patient is having. The clinic staff usually give patients literature to read about their treatment and will be happy to speak to you about practical issues, with the patient's consent.

CancerBACUP can offer advice and written information about some of the common treatments and the side effects that are commonly experienced. They can be contacted on 020 7696 9003 or their website www.cancerbacup.org.uk.

Macmillan CancerLine is a telephone service that also offers advice and information on all aspects of cancer. They can be contacted by phoning 0808 808 2020 and lines are open Monday–Friday, 9am–5pm.

More Information

The doctor and nurses are always available for advice on any aspect of practical care, so don't feel that you are on your own. The first time you tackle a new role can be quite demanding, so do not be afraid to seek advice.

A variety of agencies that can offer advice on different aspects of practical care and support for carers are listed in Appendix 4, 'Useful organisations'.

Chapter 15

The patient is requesting complementary therapy

The doctor says

Complementary therapy should be just that – complementary. It is not (in my opinion) intended to replace the role of orthodox medicine.

The older term 'alternative medicine' implied that you had a choice of 'either this or that'. The modern name 'complementary therapy' reminds us those orthodox medicines and treatments can sometimes be used in combination with complementary therapy. Because many of the agents used in complementary therapy can interfere with prescribed medications, it is essential that a suitably qualified practitioner is consulted.

I am aware that advice on complementary therapy can be obtained from a variety of sources – shops, magazines and the Internet to name but three. I cannot stress strongly enough that you must be certain that the practitioner you consult is properly qualified and registered. The appropriate professional bodies that can advise you about this are listed in Appendix 4, 'Useful organisations'.

Think

Why is the patient considering using complementary therapy?

- Is it to help them relax and maximise quality of life?
- Are they not coping with conventional treatment? Why not? Have they discussed this with the doctor?

Thinking about complementary therapies:

- Do you know the cost of the treatment being considered?
- Is it of any *proven* value?
- Is written information on complementary therapies, from reputable sources, available to you and the patient?
- Have you obtained the names of local certified practitioners?

Ask

If the patient is not tolerating or not coping with their orthodox treatment, how can you help them cope better? Complementary therapy is not a replacement for effective orthodox medicines.

Note

If the patient wishes to try complementary therapies in addition to the treatment being given by the doctors, make a note of any treatments that they are advised are safe, those that are not recommended and any other advice given with respect to their use. It is very easy to forget these details and there are so many complementary therapies that one can easily become confused.

Do ✓

Make sure that the patient complies with the treatment given by the doctor and nurses and does not stop taking any medication on the strength of starting a complementary therapy.

If a therapist suggests any change to the current treatment plan prescribed by the doctor, encourage the patient to discuss this advice with the doctor first and not to make any changes until they have had this discussion.

Explore

If the patient is interested in trying complementary therapy, make sure that they only consult practitioners who are registered with and approved by the appropriate professional body. There are unqualified persons making unfounded claims about their expertise. Appendix 4, 'Useful organisations' gives details of a selection of statutory bodies to help you.

In June 2003 the UK Nursing and Midwifery Council issued new guidelines relating to the safety of the use of complementary therapy and ensuring that therapists are appropriately trained.

More Information

Complementary therapies often involve dealing with the physical, social, psychological and spiritual aspects of a person and their illness. Patients can come away feeling that the approach is much more 'in depth' than that required by orthodox medicine and this can influence one's expectations.

The different complementary therapies vary widely in how they are administered. Some (e.g. naturopathy) offer fundamental curative treatment, while others place more emphasis on symptomatic remedies (homoeopathy).

Do not allow the patient to take any herbal remedy while on any other medication. Far from being safe to take together, they can interact – with serious side effects.

Chapter 16

The patient is confused

The doctor says

There are different mental problems that can present as confusion. To clarify the differences between them, we need some definitions.

Confusion often presents as forgetfulness and may be made worse by being in a strange environment. Impaired hearing and poor sight may compound the problem. The two main confusion syndromes seen are delirium and dementia.

Delirium is an altered state of consciousness, consisting of confusion, distractibility, disorientation, and disordered thinking and memory.

Dementia is characterised by disorientation, impaired memory, judgement and intellect, and variation in mood.

Terminal agitation is a combination of delirium and extreme anxiety sometimes seen in the last days of life.

Patients may be distressed by perfectly normal events which they misinterpret. For example, I once had a patient who was persistently trying to climb out of bed. I was asked to sedate him but, before prescribing any treatment, I asked him why he was trying to get out of bed. He replied that he 'wanted to escape from the fire'. There was no fire, but the patient in the next bed was smoking (which was allowed in those days) and the sun was shining in on his bed, making him very hot. It was a logical but incorrect interpretation of two facts – feeling heat and smelling smoke. Reassurance, removal of a blanket and finding the other patient a more suitable place to enjoy his cigarette were all that was required.

There are many possible causes of confusion, including changes in the body's chemistry with toxins building up, a brain tumour causing pressure as it grows, infection or something as simple as constipation. In the next section we'll look at these and try and help you identify the possible cause in your patient.

The doctor will need to examine the patient and possibly take blood samples to determine the cause of the confusion. In practice, confusion in terminally ill patients is often due to a combination of factors, some of which may be reversible, but some of which may persist in spite of attempts to treat them.

Think

Is the patient suffering from any of these symptoms? Tick any that you think might apply.

☐   Severe or uncontrolled pain?

☐   Constipation – especially in the elderly? (*See* Chapter 17.)

☐   A very full bladder? When did the patient last pass urine?

☐   Has the patient been coughing recently and coughing yellow or green phlegm? This could be due to a chest infection, which can cause confusion.

☐   Has the patient complained of any pain or difficulty when passing urine? An infection could be the cause of such discomfort and confusion.

☐   Is the patient suffering from a brain tumour or brain secondaries?

☐   Does the patient already suffer from Alzheimer's disease or have a history of stroke?

☐   Have the patient's medications been changed recently? An increase or decrease in certain medications could be the cause if the confusion started around the same time as changes were made.

☐   Has the patient changed (increased or decreased) their usual intake of alcohol recently?

☐   Has the confusion started since there has been a change in environment, e.g. admission to hospital or transfer from one ward to another?

Ask

Ask the doctor or nurse what is causing the confusion and what can be done to relieve the patient's distress and whether it can be treated, with a return to normal clear thinking and ability to communicate.

It is important to be aware that sometimes, near the end of the illness, the only option is to sedate the patient. Agitated or confused patients cannot really communicate, so saying your final 'goodbye' can be even more difficult than usual.

Note

Make a note of the effects of any treatment offered. Sometimes there is more than one cause for confusion and an initial improvement, followed by a worsening of the confusion, may indicate a second cause for the problem. It can be very hard to remember the exact sequence of events when asked later.

Do ✓

- Try and reduce or eliminate anything that increases anxiety and confusion – e.g. the smell of smoke if the patient thinks this indicates that the house is on fire. Confusion may be the result of correctly identified but incorrectly interpreted events.
- Don't leave the patient in the dark. Keep a light on so they can see where they are.
- Try to ensure a quiet calm atmosphere and, as far as possible, ensure that family members or other carers already known to the patient look after them.
- Prevent the patient from harming themselves and others.

Explore

While the doctors and nurses aim to involve patients in treatment decisions, most confused patients are unable to take part in this discussion.

The doctors, nurses and those caring for the patient at home, including the patient's family, must discuss and decide the best treatment options. Sometimes this can involve sedating a patient who is already quite frail. This may be the only realistic option, but carries the risk that they may then develop a chest infection by virtue of the inactivity often associated with sedation.

Speak to the doctor and other professional carers and be prepared to honestly explore and discuss the issue of sedation in such difficult circumstances.

More Information

As disease progresses, the liver and kidneys can begin to work less efficiently. Chemicals start to build up in the body and these can cause confusion. Sometimes the patient is too unwell to tolerate the treatment required to effectively treat these conditions and the only option may be to sedate the patient to relieve their distress.

By this stage of the illness, the patient may be unable to swallow tablets and the sedatives may be given by injections or by a continuous slow infusion, possibly using a syringe driver, which is a small pump about the size of a personal stereo cassette player. This is attached to a long polythene tube and a small needle which is inserted beneath the skin surface and delivers the drug over a period of time – usually 24 hours. This allows control of the symptoms with minimal disturbance of the patient.

Chapter 17

The patient is constipated

The doctor says

Most of the pain-killing drugs used for cancer cause constipation. In spite of having bran for breakfast and eating lots of fruit and vegetables, virtually every cancer patient will experience constipation. Constipation can also be due to weakness or to being less active than usual.

Strong painkillers have two effects on the bowel. First, they make it slow and sluggish. Second, they cause increased fluid loss from the bowel so the motion becomes dryer and harder.

The doctor will often prescribe a laxative at the same time as prescribing painkillers and will ask about bowel function. Because the painkiller has two effects on the bowel, two laxatives may be prescribed – one to soften the motion and one to stimulate the bowel and overcome the sluggishness caused by the painkillers. Sometimes the two types of laxatives can be given as one combined medicine. If two laxatives are prescribed, it is essential that the patient takes both. It's not an 'either/or' situation.

Patients are sometimes reluctant to talk about their bowel functions, but it is very important that the doctor knows about the problem so that they give the correct treatment. Encourage the patient to overcome their natural embarrassment: it is likely that the problem will only get worse the longer they wait. The treatment is always simplest if started early on.

Constipation is sometimes regarded as unimportant or 'normal' when we are unwell, but it makes patients uncomfortable and can cause colicky abdominal pain, loss of appetite (Chapter 12), nausea or vomiting (Chapter 31) and anxiety. In elderly patients, constipation may cause confusion (Chapter 16).

Think

Everyone has their own 'normal' bowel habit and people vary in what they regard as 'normal'. What one patient defines as 'constipation' is someone else's normal bowel habit. To make sure that they are clear about what the patient means, the doctor or nurse might ask about their use of the term 'constipation'. The nurse or doctor needs to know exactly what is 'normal' for them and how their normal bowel activity has changed.

Here are some typical questions that the doctor or nurse will ask the patient.

- What was your normal pattern of bowel action prior to your illness or starting medication?
- When did this pattern change?
- Can you associate this change with any other event, such as starting a new medication?

- When was your last normal bowel motion?
- What was its consistency?
- Have you had any pain or bleeding?
- Have you have suffered from diarrhoea (Chapter 19) or any incontinence?
- Have you bought any medicines over the counter? If so, what did you buy?

The nurse or doctor might ask about the patient's usual diet. Sometimes patients are eating less than usual or their tastes may have changed. Simple changes to diet can help, but a laxative is usually needed if the patient is taking strong painkillers. This is no reflection on the quality of your cooking!

One of the reasons people become constipated is because of a reduced fluid intake or increased fluid loss from the body – e.g. by sweating more than usual. Another way we can lose fluid is through vomiting. You might be asked about the patient's usual daily fluid intake and be advised to increase the amount of liquids they drink.

Patients in hospital can experience problems with respect to the toilet arrangements. Here are some of the things you might wish to ask the patient about.

- Is the toilet convenient?
- Is privacy adequate?
- Are you sharing one toilet with several other people and do you feel anxious about this?

Ask

If you are unsure, ask about how much fluid the patient should drink each day.

How can you increase the amount of fibre (roughage) the patient is getting?

Some laxative suspensions are very sweet. Some patients cannot tolerate sweet flavours. There are some laxative powders available that are almost tasteless and can be sprinkled on food. These might be helpful if you have alteration of normal taste (*see* Chapter 12).

Sometimes it is necessary to use two laxatives to overcome the constipation associated with strong painkillers. The patient must take both, but it might be possible for them to be given a single laxative that contains both types. Ask about this if the patient has problems with nausea or having to take too many medicines.

Note

Have you bought the patient any medication over the counter or from the pharmacist? One of the commonly sold pain-killing tablets is cocodamol (a combination of paracetamol and codeine), which is sold under a variety of trade names. Codeine is well known as a cause of constipation. Check and see if you have bought anything containing codeine and let the nurse or doctor know about this, or any other medication you purchased. You never know; it could be something as simple as that! Make a note of anything you buy for future reference.

Codeine is sometimes prescribed for an irritating cough. If the patient has been given anything for a cough, check if it contains codeine. If in doubt, ask the pharmacist.

If the patient complains of any pain or bleeding when passing a motion, make a note to remind them to discuss these with the doctor or nurse.

Do

Constipation makes people feel quite unwell and it is worth trying different ways to improve their comfort while medications and other interventions are taking effect. Sometimes massage and local heat to the abdomen provide comfort, even if they don't have any effect on the constipation. Try a heated pad or a hot water bottle wrapped in a towel, or a warm bath. Be very careful that you do not burn the patient – it's very easily done, so never use a hot water bottle that is not wrapped in a towel and never use boiling water.

Comfort measures, while they are worth trying, are not a substitute for proper advice and appropriate medication.

Explore

There are lots of advertisements in the press about 'natural ways of overcoming constipation' but many of these will not be effective and some involve taking medications that could interfere with the treatment the patient is being prescribed.

It is probably a waste of money buying laxatives from the pharmacy. Many of the products available are not strong enough. Ask the pharmacist who dispenses the patient's prescriptions so that you get the best advice. Be prepared to be advised to take the patient to see the doctor for advice and a prescription!

More Information

The doctor or nurse may wish to carry out an examination. This examination could involve pressing quite firmly over the patient's abdomen to check for areas of tenderness. This can be a little painful. It will probably be necessary to examine the back passage (rectum). This can be uncomfortable, but is important in deciding the best treatment.

Hard stools present in the rectum are usually treated by using enemas first – a small volume of fluid inserted into the back passage and sometimes left overnight to act. This may be followed by another enema of a different type the next morning. If there is difficulty in getting a good result at home, admission to hospital for a day or so is worth the fuss and bother.

After the enemas have acted, a laxative is usually given by mouth. If the laxative is given without first clearing the lower bowel, patients can develop severe crampy pain as the body tries to evacuate the hard mass of stool or will develop diarrhoea, which can be quite troublesome.

Occasionally, when there is a blockage due to hard stool higher up in the bowel, this can present as diarrhoea. This is due to the bowel content liquefying above the blockage and passing as liquid.

If the patient has bowel cancer, they need to be very careful to avoid constipation. Your aim is to keep their bowel content soft. In addition to taking laxatives as prescribed, they must have a good fluid intake and avoid non-digestible foods such as fruit peel and pith because these can cause minor blockages by forming a mesh-like network in which bowel content becomes trapped.

See the tips below for some more ideas.

Some practical tips to help avoid constipation

Constipation is almost inevitable with some of the painkillers prescribed for cancer pain unless laxatives are taken on a regular basis.

N.B. These ideas are not intended to replace any laxatives prescribed.

Exercise is helpful in getting our bodies into a routine and keeping our bowels working in a regular pattern. A gentle walk should be enough and you should encourage the patient to have some exercise each day if they feel well enough.

Fibre (roughage) is the basic essential for our bowel function. The fibre in our food allows more bulk to form in the bowel and this leads to a more regular action. Good sources of fibre include wholewheat cereals, wholemeal bread and pasta, fresh vegetables and fresh fruit with the skin kept on.

Note *Patients who are suffering from bowel cancer or who have a history of bowel obstruction should not eat fruit skins and pith.*

Grated carrot added to soup adds colour, flavour and some fibre.

Fluids are essential. Hot drinks often work best and some people find that coffee has a laxative effect. Patients suffering from constipation should drink plenty of fluids to counteract fluid loss from the bowel.

Fruit is helpful, especially if fresh or dried, with the exception of bananas, which are more likely to cause constipation than relieve it. Tinned and stewed fruit is less useful than fresh fruit.

Home remedies for constipation that have been tried and proved include prunes, prune juice and syrup of figs. Most supermarkets now stock prunes without stones, ready to eat without the need to stew them first. Prune juice is also available ready for use.

Laxatives may be necessary if these simpler measures don't work and sometimes can be helpful even when laxatives have been prescribed.

Rhubarb has been used by many people. It does not work for everyone and one of the problems is that it can be very acid and sharp. The sharp acid flavour is reduced if you stew the rhubarb in cold tea or soak it in cold tea before cooking.

Chapter 18

The patient is depressed

The doctor says

We all vary enormously in how we feel when facing difficult times. There is no 'right' or 'wrong' way to feel or to cope with the situation we are facing. One person sees the situation as a challenge to try and overcome for as long as possible, another feels threatened and just wants to give up.

Let me outline a fairly typical response over the first few weeks after being given a diagnosis of a life-threatening illness.

0–7 days

Patients commonly feel a sense of disbelief and despair and may even deny that they were told they have cancer.

7–14 days

For one to two weeks after being given bad news, patients might experience sudden changes in mood, fluctuating between feeling cheerful and positive, and feeling quite sad and 'down'.

14–21 days

After about two or three weeks the reality of the situation has usually 'sunk in'. By now the specialists have confirmed the diagnosis. At this stage patients might feel ready to start 'fighting back' and may be feeling frustration over the perceived delay in starting treatment.

I have to add that, for me, my Christian faith has been of vital importance. I believe that God will not allow anything to happen to me that is not in His plan for my life. God does not always tell us what is going on or why, but He gave me the strength to get through my first and second cancer journeys and I believe He can do so again now. I still need to plan, but I do not need to worry.

I am not alone in this thinking: the *Daily Mail* (14 August 2001)[1] reported on a research study published in the journal *Archives of Internal Medicine* showing that people with a strong faith had a better outcome to their illness.

Another paper, reviewing studies done over several decades, concludes that 'religious involvement appears to enable the sick, particularly those with serious and disabling medical illness, to cope better and experience psychological growth from their negative health experiences, rather than be defeated or overcome by them'.[2]

Another article, published in the *New Scientist*, states that those who are deeply religious are less fearful of death and that evangelicals and fundamentalists were the happiest of those surveyed.[3]

It's natural for patients to feel sad when someone tells them that they have cancer. It's possibly the worst news they has ever been given. Sadness and crying are normal responses in my opinion.

The question is, is the patient understandably sad, or are they 'clinically depressed'?

Fewer people than you might expect become 'clinically depressed'. 'Clinical depression' is a serious illness that does not go away by itself and requires treatment from the doctor. Sadness does not respond to medication – we adjust to our new circumstances and start to live our lives again, with some changes.

It's natural to be sad if someone has told you that you have cancer, but if sadness is making the patient ill, then they could be clinically depressed.

There are eight symptoms commonly associated with depression. You might wish to look at these and see how many apply to the patient.

☐	They are agitated but can't be bothered doing anything.
☐	They can't stop crying and feel low in their spirits.
☐	They feel exhausted and have no energy.
☐	They seem less interested than usual in their normal daily activities.
☐	They can't concentrate on anything.
☐	They keep thinking or talking about death.
☐	Their sleep pattern has changed (this could either be waking very early or sleeping much longer than usual).
☐	Their weight has changed (they might have gained or lost weight).

How many of the boxes did you tick? To diagnose depression, usually patients need to be suffering from at least five of the eight symptoms listed here. They are not all equally significant, nor are they listed in order of importance.

In other words, patients can feel pretty bad, but still not be 'clinically depressed' in the medical sense of the word.

Repeat this exercise again after a few days to monitor the patient's progress.

Think

There are lots of things that the patient could be worrying about and which could be contributing to their depression. Help is available for many of these problems, which may include the following:

- pain which is persistent or poorly controlled
- personal problems – particularly when we don't have the energy to deal with them
- psychological illness or depression in the past

- perceptions of the future (or lack of a future)
- personal appearance – altered by surgery or disease.

What kinds of advice or support do you think would be helpful to the patient? If you can't help and are 'out of your depth', think about using the services offered by:

- a professional counsellor
- a minister of religion or other adviser from the patient's particular faith
- a nurse or doctor – for matters relating to the illness
- a social worker – for financial and personal issues.

Ask

You might need to ask about whether the patient is suffering from:

- pain that is not under control
- the side effects of medication.

If you identify a problem that is not controlled by the current medication, ask the doctor or nurse for advice.

Note

Make a note of how the patient is behaving.

☐	Do they wake very early in the morning?
☐	How is their mood in the morning?
☐	How is their mood later in the day?
☐	Are they expressing guilt about something?
☐	Is their concentration bad?
☐	Do they not wish to speak to people, but just want to curl up and be left alone?
☐	Have they ever suffered from depression or a psychiatric illness?
☐	Are they talking about suicide or 'wishing it was all over'?
☐	Has anyone in the patient's family ever been treated for depression or a psychiatric illness?
☐	Has the patient's medication been changed recently?

Make a note of any of these issues that you need to discuss. They will help the doctor decide what needs to be done.

Do ✓

Ask for, and accept, help when you have identified the people that you think can help you and the patient. You might be surprised at the help available. For example, you do not have to be religious, or agree to a life-long commitment to a church, before a minister will offer you or the patient their support!

Encourage the patient to talk about how they feel. This might be difficult at first, but try and encourage them to 'open up', without forcing them to talk against their wishes.

Major surgery might have left the patient disfigured and feeling unattractive, incomplete, or 'less of a person than they were before'. It's not an easy subject to broach, but it needs to be discussed sooner or later. Reassure the patient that their appearance is acceptable to you.

Explore

Having cancer obviously affects one's lifestyle for a variable amount of time. The patient will probably not be able to work, so they have time to think and worry! Encourage them to take up a new hobby or interest that is not too strenuous and occupies some of their spare time.

More Information

By now, you will have realised that it can be very difficult to be sure whether patients are suffering from sadness or clinical depression. It is pointless to tell a depressed patient to 'look on the bright side' because, like Eeyore, the somewhat gloomy donkey created by AA Milne, they can't find a bright side to look on!

Sometimes the doctor will suggest a trial of an antidepressant medicine to see if it helps. This can be a useful way of confirming the diagnosis of clinical depression. It may take more than two weeks for an antidepressant drug to show any benefit, so don't give up hope after a few days because they don't seem any better.

If an antidepressant does help, it is usually given for some time. This is because, when we are depressed, essential chemicals are lost from the brain. These chemicals control our mood and it takes a few weeks to restore adequate levels. It may then be possible to gradually reduce to a lower 'maintenance' dose provided the symptoms do not return. The maintenance dose allows the body to build up its normal supplies of the chemical and allows time for recovery.

It's worth pointing out that antidepressants are not intended to make patients feel ecstatic and happy! The weakness, weariness and feeling generally unwell that are part of having cancer will still be there.

References

1 Marsh B (2001) True faith really does save lives, say doctors. *Daily Mail*. 14 August 2001.
2 Koenig HG, Larson DB and Larson SS (2001) Religion and coping with serious medical illness. *Annals of Pharmacotherapeutics*. **35**(3): 352–9.
3 Bond M (2003) Feelgood factor: part 1 – the pursuit of happiness. *New Scientist*. **180**(2415): 40–47.

Chapter 19

The patient has diarrhoea

The doctor says

Diarrhoea is not usually as common as constipation (*see* Chapter 17) among cancer patients, but there are exceptions to every rule. Cancer patients can still get tummy upsets and food poisoning just like anyone else. Some patients might even be more prone to diarrhoea if their immune system is not working as well as normal because of the treatment. If this is the case, they will have been advised to be extra careful about cooking food thoroughly, not reheating food, avoiding fast food restaurants and also checking 'best before' dates and avoiding anything that is past its sell-by date.

Radiotherapy to the abdomen or pelvis can result in some diarrhoea. The staff will give advice about how long it might last.

Patients who have had surgery to the bowel, particularly those who have had part of the bowel removed, can suffer from diarrhoea as a result. After bowel surgery, one's tolerance of various foods, especially fruit and vegetables, might have changed.

Ulcerative colitis and Crohn's disease both cause diarrhoea but sufferers from these diseases will be well aware of that already.

Some medicines and tablets, including some chemotherapy drugs, can cause diarrhoea. Finally, as I mentioned in Chapter 17, severe constipation can cause diarrhoea.

Think

Think about these and tick anything that applies.

☐	How long has the patient had diarrhoea?
☐	Had the patient been constipated immediately before the diarrhoea started?
☐	Did the patient's diarrhoea begin after starting on a new medicine or tablets?
☐	Has the patient had radiotherapy to their abdomen recently?
☐	Has the patient started taking laxatives for the first time, changed their laxative or changed the dose of their usual laxative?
☐	Is anyone else in the family affected? If so, it might be a 'tummy bug' that is responsible.

The doctor will use this information to decide the likely cause of the problem.

Ask

If the diarrhoea started immediately after a change in the patient's medication, ask if it might be the cause of their diarrhoea. Find out if this is a known side effect and how long it is likely to persist. An alternative treatment might be available.

Diarrhoea that starts following bowel surgery might be persistent. You might want to ask about what foods to avoid, but often this is a matter of 'trial and error' because people react quite differently to different foods.

Note

Make a note of any changes in treatment that you think might be responsible for the patient's diarrhoea and ask about these.

Keep a record of any foods that seem to upset the patient. In general, fruit and certain vegetables are common culprits but other foods, such as cream or a white sauce for fish, upset some people but not others.

Do

- Encourage the patient to drink plenty of fluids to make up for the fluid they are losing from their bowels. Try to avoid giving fruit juices and sugary drinks as these are likely to make things worse.
- Avoid serving fruit, vegetables and high fibre foods until things settle. Re-introduce them in small portions at first, one at a time, making a note of any that don't suit.
- Ask about whether any prescribed laxative should be temporarily stopped or given in reduced doses.
- Make sure the patient continues to take all medications as instructed. Ask about any that seem to upset them and seek appropriate advice about how to manage this.

Explore

There really is not much to explore on this topic! There are plenty of remedies that you can buy from the pharmacy for diarrhoea, but before you do buy anything, tell the pharmacist what treatment the patient is taking so that anything you might buy will not interfere with something being prescribed.

More Information

The nurse or doctor will want to conduct an examination to find the cause and decide how to treat the diarrhoea. This is likely to involve:

- an abdominal examination
- examination of the patient's rectum (back passage) to exclude constipation. If the lower bowel is congested, the stools above can liquefy and drain away as diarrhoea.

The doctor may request a stool sample for examination in the laboratory if a bowel infection is suspected.

Very occasionally, blood tests might be required.

Chapter 20

The patient is not drinking enough

The doctor says

We all need to drink plenty of fluids when we are ill. Our fluid losses can increase as we lie in bed because we tend to sweat slightly more and we need to counteract these 'insensible losses'. Fluid loss due to sweating increases dramatically during any infection, so increasing one's intake of fluids should be encouraged if infection is present or suspected – e.g. if the patient has a raised temperature.

Patients might not wish to drink for a variety of reasons. These include weakness, loss of interest in food and fluids, altered taste and simply the fact that drinking more means extra trips to the bathroom, which are exhausting.

Altered taste can make eating and drinking most unpalatable. I was unable to drink water for several weeks because of altered taste due to chemotherapy. I was sick after drinking water several times and quite simply had to find something I could keep down. This was a case of 'trial and error' until I found a palatable drink. What I did find was that if drinks were very cold I could tolerate them better.

Think

Are you aware of why the patient might not be drinking enough? For example, have they complained of any of the following:

- Altered taste of food and water?
- Feeling sick when eating or drinking?
- Feeling full and unable to drink?
- Tiredness so that they wish to avoid extra trips to the bathroom?
- Does the patient need your help to get to the bathroom? Do they think you can't cope with this extra work?

Ask

Ask the patient why they don't wish to drink. If there is no specific reason given, try to encourage them to drink more to overcome the fluid losses that are associated with being in bed and sweating more than usual.

Note

Make a note of any specific reason why the patient does not wish to drink. Do you need to discuss these with the doctor or nurse?

Do ✓

Try new drinks. It is worth trying the isotonic 'sports' drinks too, as these are sometimes better tolerated than water or diluted fruit juice drinks. Many patients develop an aversion to tea and coffee after chemotherapy. My intake of tea decreased from multiple cups per day to nil for several weeks! Try other drinks e.g. 'Bovril' or cup soups but buy small jars initially in case you end up with a shelf of unused products!

Frail patients who are less able to drink may suffer from a dry mouth (*see* Chapter 26). You can help in several ways such as offering pieces of ice to suck, regular sips of cold water or even small amounts of water dripped from a syringe into the patient's mouth if they are very frail.

Patients who have a dry mouth are especially prone to thrush infection, which shows up as red areas, possibly with white patches, and is painful. This needs to be treated by the doctor and will not clear up by itself.

Explore

If the reason for not drinking enough is because the patient does not wish to have to use the bathroom, explore the possibility of obtaining a urinal for men or a commode for women patients.

Commodes take up space, can compromise privacy and are hard to disguise, so they can draw attention to the fact that the patient is getting weaker. Discuss the provision of these items with the community nurse. Sometimes the Red Cross can offer these items on short-term loan.

More Information 📖

It's not common for patients at home to have a drip put up, but it occasionally happens. Before asking about intravenous fluids (a drip), think about the following issues associated with this type of treatment.

Many patients and relatives believe that an intravenous drip provides adequate nutrition. There is little evidence to suggest that simple fluids achieve this. Adequate nutrition by means of a drip in the vein usually requires hospital admission and expert advice.

If an intravenous drip is requested, especially in a seriously ill patient, there can be several consequences. These include the following possibilities:

- care at home may not be possible
- an increase in urine output means more trips to the bathroom (will the patient need a catheter?)
- increased secretions (may increase cough and vomiting).

A strange, but true, consequence in the very poorly patient is that increased fluid intake can increase their awareness of discomfort and pain. This is because the increased fluid intake washes out certain chemicals that had been making the patient a bit drowsy and less aware of their pain and general discomfort. Sometimes it is kinder to allow some degree of drowsiness and lack of awareness of pain. This decision is best made by the doctor and nurse, so let them guide you.

Chapter 21

The patient needs equipment to assist with day-to-day care

The doctor says

Over the years, I have lost count of the number of people who have said to me that they could have coped much more easily if they had known of the existence of a particular device or piece of equipment.

The number of aids available is increasing all the time and availability is much easier than it was a few years ago. I cannot possibly hope to do more than raise awareness and advise you to ask the doctor or occupational therapist, who can advise about specific needs and how they can be met.

Think

What difficulties are you and/or the patient facing? Are these problems the result of their current illness or treatment?

When do the difficulties arise, is it with:

- Eating and drinking?
- Getting in and out of bed?
- Getting to and from the toilet?
- Bathing?
- Needing help at night but you don't hear when you are called?

These are only suggestions. You need to sit and think about the patient's needs and compile your own list.

Ask

Ask yourself

- What equipment do you think would help you cope more easily with the tasks that you find difficult?
- Who can help you obtain this equipment?
- Do you feel confident to use this equipment and how do you think the equipment will help you?

Ask the patient

- What activities or tasks do they find difficult, even with your help?
- How do they think the task could be made easier?

- Are they confident to allow you to continue to care for them and use the equipment?

Note

Make a note of any problems you anticipate, any anxieties expressed by the patient and any demonstrations or training you might need to be able to use an item you borrow.

Make a note of the person you should contact if you experience problems using any equipment you obtain.

Do ✔

Only agree to undertake the continuing care of the patient if you are absolutely sure that you can cope with their needs. Using equipment can be an added skill to acquire, not a guarantee that it will make life problem-free!

Ensure that you have room for anything you borrow or hire – a hospital bed and a hoist may require more floor space than you have available. The size of your doors may dictate what can be used in your home, so be prepared to do some preparatory measuring and possibly to have to sacrifice a favourite armchair for a while!

Remember, it may be difficult or impossible to have heavy or bulky equipment taken upstairs. Is it easier to bring the bed downstairs? What about access to the toilet? Effective care needs careful planning.

Explore

Spend some time finding out what kinds of equipment are available. Here are a few of the commoner items.

Bath aids

Bathing can present a real problem and you must remember the risk of injury to the patient and yourself. It's easy to slip, over-reach or hurt your back trying to prevent injury to the patient, so be realistic about what you can do regarding bathing.

Having said this, grab rails, seats, bath mats and other appliances are available. Grab rails and other items must be properly fitted and it is best to seek expert advice because the risk of injury is quite substantial if these items are not securely fixed in position.

Bedpans and bottles

Urine bottles with non-spill valves are relatively cheap and easy to get. Bedpans are also easily available and they can make life easier by reducing the number of trips to the bathroom.

Bed-raisers

A couple of bricks, left over from the time you built a barbecue in the garden, are *not* suitable for raising the bed or a chair! They can very easily slip and it's just not worth the risk. Specially designed bed and chair raisers are readily available, usually from the occupational therapist, and are safe. These give the added height that can make sitting and standing much easier.

Commodes and toilet-seat raisers

Commodes and plastic devices to raise the toilet seat by 3–4 inches can usually be borrowed. Ask the community nurse about these. They can be purchased if you prefer.

Commodes are difficult to disguise! Their presence draws attention to the patient's reduced ability to get to and from the bathroom and they may be the cause of some embarrassment and upset. It is also important to remember the need for adequate privacy if a commode is required.

Free-standing metal frames that fit round the toilet to assist with sitting and standing are also available. Before one is ordered, it is essential to accurately measure the space available to ensure that the frame chosen will fit.

Cutlery and crockery

Heated plates to prevent food getting cold if one eats slowly, raised edges for the plate to prevent food being pushed off and specially shaped cups are available to help with eating and drinking.

Cutlery with chunky soft-grip handles helps those with a poor grip, and specially shaped forks and spoons can help if one has difficulty with feeding.

Many of these can be bought from larger chemists or shops that sell equipment for disabled persons at very reasonable prices and most are dishwasher-safe. Another possible source is the 'independent living catalogue' available from Lloyds chemists.

Handrails

Handrails can be fitted near a door, near steps or near a bath or toilet as required. The occupational therapist can order them or you can buy and fit them yourself.

The important thing is that if you decide to fit these yourself, make sure that they will support the patient's weight. In a modern timber-framed home with plasterboard walls they must be fitted to the wooden battens in the framework behind the plasterboard for adequate support. If in doubt, ask a skilled person to do this for you.

Hoists

Hoists are used for lifting patients into and out of the bath or bed. My personal view is that you need to be trained in how to use a hoist, that the hoist must be chosen by a competent, trained person and it must meet the patient's individual needs.

Mattresses

Skin care is of the utmost importance and the type of mattress used can have a very significant effect on skin care and vulnerability.

Mattresses come in all types, from basic egg-box design to fully remote controlled air-beds. A nurse who is trained and experienced in this type of care must assess the needs of the individual patient. I do not recommend that you try to pick a mattress out of a glossy magazine or be persuaded to buy something because a salesperson recommends it.

Ramps

Ramps to allow easier wheelchair access can be bought but it is often better to have them 'made to measure' to allow adequate width and a slope that is not too steep.

Two-way listeners

Listening devices, of the type usually advertised for use with babies, provide a simple and reliable method of keeping in touch while getting on with other duties around the house. Some can be plugged in and run off the mains; others are portable and battery operated, which means they can be clipped to a belt or pocket.

Wheelchairs

For short-term use, wheelchairs can often be borrowed from the local supplies department (ask the community nurse) or from the Red Cross. The GP can request a wheelchair for longer-term use.

Of equal importance is the cushion and support offered by the wheelchair. The patient's skin can be put at risk by an unsuitable chair. If in doubt, ask for expert advice.

If the patient wishes to buy their own wheelchair, it is essential that a trained person measures them for their chair. This is the only way to ensure that the appropriate chair is chosen.

More Information

It will be clear by now that I am wary of people buying equipment without first seeking expert guidance. Always remember that salespeople may be driven by the commission paid to them on the sale of a particular item and may not be trained to fully assess the needs of the patient.

The NHS covers most needs. If you choose to buy, that's fair enough, but do ask the nurse, doctor or occupational therapist for advice before buying an expensive piece of equipment, only to find that it does not suit.

If you do 'buy and try', make sure that you have, in writing, a guarantee of a full refund if you need to return an unsuitable item after a reasonable trial.

Finally, do remember that if you borrowed equipment that the patient is no longer using, return it promptly. Someone else is struggling while they await the availability of the item stored in the patient's garage!

Chapter 22

The patient has a fistula

The doctor says

If you don't understand the term 'fistula', then you can probably ignore this chapter! However, in case you are curious, I'll explain myself. A favourite question when I was a medical student was 'What is the difference between a fistula and a sinus?'

A *fistula* is an abnormal passage or opening from one surface to another surface. They may form between two internal organs or between an internal organ and the skin surface. The word 'fistula' comes from the Latin word for pipe or tube. Fistulas may therefore form an abnormal passage between two internal organs or may allow leakage to the outside.

A *sinus* is a cavity or hollow space. In other words, it is a blind cul-de-sac. It originates from the Latin word for a hollow.

Fistulas are not very common. Only about 1% of patients with advanced cancer will develop a fistula and they are commonest in bowel cancer or after radiotherapy to the pelvic area.

Basically a fistula forms either when the cancer progresses through the surface of one organ into another – e.g. from the rectum (back passage) into the vagina, or when the diseased tissues are further damaged by radiotherapy in a tumour that does not respond to this treatment.

Fistulas are very distressing but there are things that can be done to help you manage the difficulties they present.

Think

There are several problems associated with fistulas, each of which is difficult to deal with and distressing. You might agree with some of these comments that have been made by other carers:

- The appearance of the fistula distresses the patient and me.
- I think the patient feels that having a fistula makes them unattractive and unacceptable to me.
- The fistula leaks an offensive-smelling liquid.
- I think the patient is afraid of being socially unacceptable.

Ask

Fistulas need to be managed according to the patient's individual needs, so do not be afraid to ask for advice and help. Ask for a specialist nurse to see the patient because they have greater experience and expertise in these problems and can offer the best advice.

If the fistula is leaking out onto the skin, ask about dressings or whether an adhesive bag is available to absorb the leaking fluid. The persistent dampness of the skin may make it difficult to find a suitable adhesive.

If the fistula is leaking bowel content to the skin, some odour will occur. Ask what can be done to minimise it. As a rule, 'air fresheners' are a waste of time and sometimes only draw attention to the fact that there is a problem!

Report any redness or soreness of the skin to the nurse or doctor early on. There are ways of protecting the skin against the effects of being moist and becoming sore. Pain may be due to infection and, if so, this is usually easy to treat. Report problems early because they won't get better on their own.

Note

There are likely to be different people involved in caring for the patient's fistula, so it might help for you to make a note of their names, what they do and how to contact them if there are any problems that you can't manage.

Make a note of the treatments and ideas that help and those that do not. This will help prevent you re-trying ideas that are not effective.

Do ✓

Depending on the site of the patient's fistula, there are practical ideas that might be worth trying. I have listed some of the commoner sites and some suggestions that have helped other patients.

Fistulas of the mouth

The constant leakage of saliva and of food is distressing and can affect one's general health. The constant moistness may make the skin round the mouth prone to becoming sore and breaking down.

A simple plug of clean gauze may seal off a small fistula, absorbing the excess saliva and allowing the patient to eat more easily.

If the constant dribbling of saliva is a problem, ask the doctor about tablets to reduce the amount of saliva produced. This carries the risk of developing a dry mouth (*see* Chapter 26). The patient must decide which is more acceptable. It's always worth a try.

A fistula between the bowel and the skin surface

These can produce a large amount of fluid or more solid bowel content. Trying to contain this with a simple absorbent dressing rarely works.

A colostomy bag, fitted over the opening, may help collect the effluent when a fistula develops between the bowel and the abdominal wall. The stoma nurse will be able to give very valuable advice on skin protection and the most suitable type of bag.

Patients who have had a lot of surgery and have a very scarred tummy with an uneven surface might think that there is no way a bag will fit without leaking. Special skin fillers can be used to create a smooth even surface to overcome this problem. Ask the stoma nurse about this.

Various ideas can be tried to control odour and the stoma nurse will help you find the one that is best.

A fistula between the rectum and vagina

This is a very distressing problem for any woman. Talk to the nurse or doctor about whether it would help to try and make the stool firmer by:

- reducing the dose of any prescribed laxatives
- being prescribed something to make the stool firmer.

Vaginal tampons may also help to absorb excess fluid. Use a tampon that expands horizontally rather than vertically (e.g. Lil-lets).

Ask the nurse or doctor about the patient's personal hygiene and ways to reduce the risk of infection.

If the patient is well enough, they might be offered an operation to form a colostomy (an artificial opening of the bowel to the surface of the abdomen, with a bag to collect the bowel content). This could give relief, if the patient is fit for an operation.

A fistula between the bladder and rectum

In this event, bowel content leaks into the bladder or urine leaks into the rectum. Either way, the result is very unpleasant. Surgery is the best option, if it is feasible and acceptable. Otherwise, attention to hygiene and keeping the bowel content reasonably firm and manageable are the main things to do.

A fistula between the bladder and vagina

Surgery to create a urinary diversion can bring complete relief. Otherwise, try to absorb excess fluid by use of tampons and reminding the patient to empty their bladder regularly.

Explore

Do enquire about new techniques and treatments, but don't rush into trying anything you see advertised without asking the nurse or doctor first.

To be honest, I have not seen anything advertised that I could recommend for the patient to try.

More Information

Sometimes the smell of a fistula is due to infection and this can be controlled by use of antibiotics.

A variety of treatments might be discussed and this is more likely if several professionals are involved. Not every treatment discussed will be suitable, so don't be too disappointed if ideas are suggested but not put into action. On the other hand, new treatments are becoming available all the time, so don't be afraid to ask.

Chapter 23

The patient needs to get out and about more

The doctor says

Over the 25 years that I've been a doctor, many relatives have expressed their concerns about patients not getting enough exercise and spending too much time indoors.

It's easy to look out at a lovely sunny day and think that it's too good to waste indoors and I'd be among the first to think that way. A few years ago, however, I remember spending several lovely sunny days lying in my bed, duvet up to my chin and with the cat lying on top of me, with no interest or desire to go out. In case you wonder, we didn't encourage the cat to sleep on our bed, but he had come to find me and I was feeling too unwell to tell him off!

Think

- Does the patient usually enjoy being out of doors?
- Is the patient able to manage steps and stairs?
- Does the patient get short of breath on exercise?

Some people prefer being inside with a window open. Being short of breath or feeling weak can be a deterrent to anyone who normally enjoys fresh air and the slightest hill can seem like a mountain when one is breathless.

Ask

Ask the patient if they would like to go outside. If they would, find out if there are any practical issues that might present a problem and try to find ways to overcome these. If walking is a problem or breathlessness limits their exercise tolerance, think about borrowing a wheelchair and a portable ramp if necessary. *See* Chapter 21 'The patient needs equipment to assist with day-to-day care' for more details.

Note

After a trial of getting out, make a note of any problems encountered, how these might be resolved and any problems that you need to deal with if you decide to repeat this exercise.

Do ✔

Take on a short walk the first time. Remember that wherever you go, you have also got to come back and it's the last bit of the journey that's always the most demanding.

If you are going out by car, find out about parking and the location of essential facilities such as toilets. They are not always placed at the locations most easily accessed by someone who is feeling weak or short of breath!

Visits to shops are much easier if they are not crowded. I developed a hatred of being in busy stuffy shops and found it much easier to get up early and be finished with my main shopping before the crowds arrived. Alice is now finding the same thing.

Do the most strenuous and demanding things first when the patient is fresh and feels stronger. Take time for a coffee break and finish with the things that you find most enjoyable, or least strenuous and stressful.

Explore

Look for places that are easily accessed, not too hilly for a breathless or tired patient and that have plenty of places to sit and rest. We used to go out for lunch and then sit on a canal bank a short walk away and feed the swans. It sounds terribly basic, but it allowed us to be in the fresh air, was not too exhausting and we both enjoyed it.

Think about a disabled person's badge for the car. The rules are quite specific – one must be permanently and substantially disabled, but it is worth asking.

National Rail has special facilities for disabled passengers. It might be worth picking up their booklet *Rail Travel for Disabled Passengers*, which includes an application form for a Disabled Persons Railcard. Alternatively, there is a Helpline on 0191 218 8103 and a textphone for those with hearing difficulties on 0191 269 0304. To qualify for a Disabled Persons Railcard, the patient must be registered disabled, be blind or deaf, or be in receipt of Attendance Allowance or Disability Living Allowance.

Find a pleasant country site, a seaside spot or a park where you can relax.

More Information 📖

Even the sunniest warmest day might not be enough for the patient to muster up the energy to go out. The weakness of illness, the anaemia and exhaustion associated with chemotherapy and radiotherapy treatment can be so debilitating that the very thought of having to put on shoes and a jacket can be too much.

Alice and I certainly felt very frustrated some days as we saw the summer pass and both felt too unwell to enjoy it.

Don't hassle the patient. Plan and suggest something very simple. Sometimes the fear of not being able to achieve the goal is quite overwhelming. A comfortable seat in the garden, even for a few minutes, might be enough to start with.

Chapter 24

The patient is jaundiced

The doctor says

'Jaundice' is a description, not a disease. The word is actually derived from an old French word meaning 'yellow coloured'.

Jaundice causes yellowing of the skin and the whites of the eyes. The patient's urine becomes dark and bowel motions become pale.

There are many possible causes for jaundice. They may be completely unrelated to the patient's current illness. Some causes of jaundice are:

- gallstones
- hepatitis (inflammation of the liver due to infection or toxins)
- pancreatitis (inflammation of the pancreas)
- some medicines, though you should have been made aware if this was thought to be likely.

Think

In order to offer the correct treatment, the exact cause of jaundice must be established. Alcohol and infections spread by sharing needles to inject drugs are among the possible causes these days. No offence is intended by enquiring into these possibilities. The fact is, the doctor simply needs to know. If there is a possibility of an infectious cause, the blood samples are infectious too and the laboratory staff must be warned. Please do not be offended by the questions I am inviting you to think about. The simple fact is, in the 21st century, the 'lifestyle questions' are relevant.

- Has the patient ever had a blood transfusion?
- Has the patient ever had jaundice before? If so, when, and how was it treated?
- Has the patient any pain, particularly in the upper abdomen?
- Has the patient been itching?
- How much alcohol does the patient drink?
- Has the patient ever been abroad? If so, where and when?
- Has the patient suffered any illness (with or without jaundice) at the time of that trip?
- Has the patient had vaccines to protect against hepatitis?
- Has the patient ever had an injection given outwith the UK?
- Has the patient ever, at any time, shared a needle to inject drugs?

Ask

You may wish to ask about the cause of the patient's jaundice and how it can be treated. You might also want to know about the various tests being ordered and how they help in assessing the cause and most effective treatment. Don't forget that the doctor or nurse can only discuss these matters with you if the patient agrees.

Note

Jaundiced patients can be very unwell, so you might need to make a note of any treatment offered and how effective it is. Record any side effects to report to the nurse or doctor.

Do ☑

Make sure the patient gets plenty of rest, eats a healthy diet, takes the treatment prescribed and avoids alcohol.

Do not buy any medicine or give any medicine without asking for advice first.

Explore

On the basis of unfortunate, expensive and time-wasting experiences of others, I would advise extreme caution in exploring any course of action not recommended by the doctor.

Do not be deceived into thinking that some complementary treatments, e.g. herbal remedies, are 'harmless'. This is not always the case, as others have found out! The fact is, many are not fully researched, contain much more complex chemicals than one might think and can interfere with prescribed medication or may be unsuitable for the patient.

More Information 📖

Jaundice can be the sign of progressing disease causing increasing damage to the liver. Sometimes there is nothing that can be done to halt this process. If this is the case, which can often be determined by simple blood tests, the doctor may consider that scans and biopsies will add no new information and therefore may not order these tests.

As the disease progresses, the changes in skin colour can develop and change very rapidly. This can be alarming, especially to younger members of the family.

Chapter 25

The patient has lymphoedema

The doctor says

Let's start with a few definitions to explain what lymphoedema is.

Lymph is a fluid that is collected from the tissues throughout the body, and is returned, via the lymph nodes, to the blood. The Latin word 'lympha' means 'clear spring water'.

Oedema (sometimes spelled edema) is an accumulation of watery fluid in the tissues. It is commonly seen around the ankles of elderly people.

The word 'lymphoedema' is made up from these two words. Lymphoedema is the accumulation of lymph just under the surface of the skin. It causes swelling and thickening of the skin around affected areas. Usually one limb is affected, becoming swollen, heavy, tight and uncomfortable. The whole limb (arm or leg) tends to be affected. Simple oedema usually affects both ankles.

What does lymph do?

Basically, in order to nourish the deeper tissues in our bodies, some fluid oozes out of our blood vessels, carrying food to the tissues where even the smallest blood vessels cannot reach.

After giving up nutrients, the fluid absorbs any waste products in the tissues and is reabsorbed into lymph channels and pumped back to rejoin the blood circulation and have waste products removed and new nutrients added for the next journey. On the way back to the blood stream, the lymph passes through the 'lymph nodes' which are a series of filters, situated throughout your body, but especially in the groins, under the arms and in your neck. Anything that could damage the body is trapped in these lymph nodes and the body then tries to destroy them. That's why you get 'swollen glands' during an infection – the lymph nodes are full of white blood cells which have captured germs that being are filtered out and destroyed.

What causes lymphoedema?

Lymph drains from the distant parts back towards the heart, so it flows through lymph nodes in your groins and under your arms on its way back. If the lymph nodes are permanently damaged, either because they were removed, have been damaged by disease, surgery or radiotherapy, or are blocked because they have trapped cancer cells which are now growing there, the lymph can't flow freely and the affected limb swells. Usually only one side of the body is affected.

Think

Patients suffering from lymphoedema usually are cared for by more than one professional, so you might be required to take the patient to several clinics. The effective management of lymphoedema can be quite complicated because lymphoedema can affect the patient's life in a number of ways. Here are some of the common problems associated with a swollen limb affected by lymphoedema.

- Difficulty in bending the arm or leg.
- Difficulty putting on or taking off shoes, socks, etc.
- Difficulty with putting on clothes – e.g. fastening buttons. Clothes may become tight round the arms or legs as fluid gathers during the day.
- The arm or leg may feel 'heavy'.
- The patient may have difficulty moving around the house, climbing the stairs or getting into bed.
- The patient may experience difficulty having a bath or shower.
- General household tasks, e.g. working in the kitchen, can pose a risk. There is a risk of cuts and grazes to the affected arm and the patient might find it difficult to hold kitchen items.
- The patient may find it difficult or impossible to carry out routine tasks unaided due to the swelling, tightness or pain in the limb.

Be aware of these possibilities. What can you do to help? What tasks will you find difficult? For example, can you help with washing, dressing and getting into and out of bed? You are allowed to have 'boundaries' and if you cannot help with certain aspects of the patient's care, this needs to be fully discussed with the patient and the other carers.

Ask

It is worthwhile to discuss the problem(s) the patient is experiencing and to ask about adaptations to clothes, provision of aids to help with daily living or with working in the house. Here are some of the items that might help the patient maintain their independence or make life easier.

- Long-handled devices are available for picking things up from the floor.
- Adaptations can be made to clothes – buttons can be replaced with velcro and sleeves can be made wider and loose.
- Sometimes a specially designed pocket or apron can be made to support a swollen arm.
- Various aids are available to help patients work one-handed and reduce the risk of cuts and grazes to the affected limb.
- If the patient's leg is badly swollen, it may be appropriate to ask about powered bath hoists and powered recliner/self-lift chairs to help maintain independence. Do not try to choose these items yourself.

The patient may be assessed by a physiotherapist, or a lymphoedema nurse specialist. The patient might have to travel to a specialist centre to be seen but the trip will be well worth the effort.

Note

Make a note of any activities that seem to make the swelling become worse or more painful. Can you help the patient with any of these? Here are some changes that you might note in the patient's skin in the affected limb.

- Redness, heat or pain (ask about pain).
- Breaks in the skin around the affected area. (A small break in the skin could allow an infection to start.)
- Leakage of fluid through breaks in the skin. This may be noted on clothing or bed linen.
- Ulcers or weeping areas on the affected skin.

Do

Encourage the patient to keep the swollen limb raised to assist drainage of fluid back into the body. Fluid always runs down the hill!

Provide enough pillows that the patient can raise their arm to the height of their shoulder. Avoid rough fabric that could hurt the skin. Pillow covers are usually a suitable and easy option.

When sitting, patients with a swollen leg should keep their legs up, at least level with their hips. The foot of the bed can be raised at night by 2–3 inches. Do not use bricks, because they can slip. Specially designed 'bed-raisers' are available and must be securely fitted.

If you are assisting the patient with washing, always dry well between their fingers and toes. Use a hair drier at the lowest heat setting if you have difficulty getting a towel between the swollen toes or fingers and don't forget, the skin is easily damaged.

If you see any signs of inflammation (redness, pain and heat) ask for advice and treatment from the doctor promptly. Infection can spread rapidly and needs an antibiotic.

Explore

A swollen limb is unpleasant and it is tempting to seek advice over the Internet and from other sources. Knowing others who have suffered and not benefited as a result of such explorations, my personal opinion is that the patient should let the professionals continue to advise about appropriate treatment.

More Information

If the patient has a dressing on their swollen limb because it leaks fluid, the dressing will be much more easily removed if well soaked in sterile saline (salt) solution. The nurse will provide the sterile saline or advise you about other methods of loosening the dressing. Do not make up your own solution at home – use sterile saline. Do not attempt to remove a dressing that is stuck to the skin without soaking it first.

There are several specialist techniques used to control swelling of arms and legs. You might hear about them and wonder what is involved, so here are a few common ones. At risk of repeating myself: these are specialist techniques – do not be tempted to try and do any of these for the patient.

- **Compression bandaging**: This is a special technique involving bandaging from fingers/toes up the whole limb. Layers of cotton wool and stretchy bandages are used to give more compression at the fingers and toes and less at the top of the limb. A specially trained nurse or physiotherapist will do this.
- **Compression stockings and sleeves**: These may be made-to-measure and they work by prevent fluid accumulating and giving firm support. They are designed so that the pressure is graduated, i.e. highest at the hand or foot. Do not attempt to buy a sleeve or a 'support stocking' from a catalogue or over the counter. Accurate measurements are the only way to ensure a properly fitted sleeve or stocking that is suited to the individual patient's needs.
- **Massage**: This is certainly not the kind of massage you have after a sauna! It's a special technique, very gently massaging the tissues to encourage the lymph to flow through the swollen lymph nodes and back into the body.
- **Intermittent compression pumps**: These are of limited value. They have a role in some situations, but choosing such devices is the work of highly trained professionals. Don't even be tempted to try and choose one.

Finally, it is natural and normal for patients to feel distress and to be upset because of their swollen deformed limb. Be prepared for emotional upsets and changes of mood.

Chapter 26

The patient's mouth is dry

The doctor says

Actually, I have asked a dentist to offer her input to this and the next chapter, so this section really should be headed 'The dentist says'!

Having a dry mouth is a nuisance, but there is much more to it than just nuisance value. Saliva has several functions including:

- Keeping our mouths moist, allowing our lips and tongue to move around without getting stuck to the roof of our mouth and our teeth. Saliva also helps to provide a slight suction, which helps to hold a denture in place.
- Allowing us to speak clearly.
- Adding calcium to our teeth. Calcium is essential for healthy teeth, helping to reduce decay, especially round the margins of our gums, which become very vulnerable if our mouths are dry.
- Moistening and softening our food and helping us to appreciate its taste.
- Neutralising the acids that form in our mouths after we eat food. These acids attack the enamel surfaces of the teeth, then bacteria cause decay in the damaged surfaces.
- An antiseptic action that helps to kill the bacteria that cause decay.

So, a dry mouth is much more than a nuisance. The patient's teeth are at risk. Keeping dentures in place in a dry mouth can be a major problem. Dentures can cause small cuts, and these can become infected if we don't take care. This is dealt with in Chapter 27 'The patient's mouth is sore'.

Think

The risk to one's teeth increases in proportion to how long the dry mouth persists. If possible, patients should see a dentist early on. They will need to know:

- How long has the patient suffered from a dry mouth?
- Did it start suddenly, or develop slowly over a period of time?

Various medical conditions and some treatments can make the mouth dry. For example:

- poorly controlled diabetes
- certain medications – some that may cause a dry mouth include antihistamines for allergy, anticonvulsants for fits, beta-blockers for high blood pressure, diuretics for fluid retention, some antidepressants, and some strong painkillers
- mouth infections e.g. thrush (candida)
- reduced fluid intake – possibly due to feeling sick

- radiotherapy to the head and neck can cause reduced saliva production
- use of oxygen to help one's breathing – oxygen is very dry, even if bubbled through a water chamber to try to add some moisture
- mouth-breathing when asleep – patients who mouth-breathe while sleeping usually waken up with a very dry mouth, sometimes with a bad taste in their mouth.

Ask

There are a number of ways you can help the patient reduce their risk of tooth decay.

- Enquire about the use of a fluoride mouthwash.
- Ask about a fluoride gel that they can use at night when the risk is greatest.
- Ask about how often they should see the dentist or hygienist. Since there is the risk of more rapid tooth decay, it makes sense to be seen more frequently to deal with problems early on. If the patient is immobile, most dentists will visit at home to assess and advise.

Note

While some fruits are very bland and pleasant to eat, others that you find quite palatable can be 'sharp' to the patient whose mouth is dry. Most patients experience altered taste when their mouths are dry and this might change with time.

Keep a note of the things the patient can enjoy and can eat without discomfort.

Do

Encourage the patient to drink plenty of fluids. Our mouths can become dry if our bodies are even slightly dehydrated.

Even if patients are drinking plenty of fluids, certain conditions – e.g. radiotherapy – result in damage to the salivary glands that means that the patient's mouth will become dry anyway. One way to overcome this is to carry a small bottle of water to sip frequently. So many people carry and drink bottled water these days that the patient will not look out of place.

Driving can be a bit of a problem. Drinking from a bottle involves putting your head back and losing sight of the road for a moment. I overcame this by a 'drinks holder' hung on the window of the driver's door. I also found a child's drink bottle with a plastic straw in the lid fitted perfectly. I can sip through the straw and still watch the road. If the patient is driving, or even a passenger, this is worth trying.

Sucking ice cubes or frozen fruit segments, e.g. orange or pineapple (fresh, or tinned in natural juice – not syrup), can freshen the mouth. Pineapple is also effective in clearing away any sticky debris that gathers on the patient's tongue. It is acidic, so offer the patient a drink of water afterwards to protect their teeth from the acid.

If the patient wakens up with a sticky mouth, try a mouthwash of sodium bicarbonate (1 teaspoon in a pint of warm water) as a mouthwash but *they should not swallow it*. This is an excellent and cheap mouthwash for a sore mouth, e.g. during chemotherapy and radiotherapy.

If you see signs of infection with sore or red areas, with or without white spots, ask the doctor or dentist for treatment. It could be thrush infection and will not clear up on its own.

Dentures must be kept meticulously clean. Dentures harbour tiny particles of food and these are an ideal medium for growing infection. Advise the patient to remove their dentures at night unless the dentist has advised otherwise. If the patient wears an obturator following maxillofacial surgery, ask for specialist advice if they are having problems with recurring soreness or infection.

Oral hygiene is very important. If at all possible the patient should see their dentist before starting treatment such as radiotherapy. I know they will not want to be bothered, but it is much better to start treatment with a clean bill of (dental) health and be given expert advice, than to wait until they feel up to it and get round to making an appointment after the treatment has finished. Any dental work needing to be done before starting treatment will be easier on them physically, and probably cheaper!

Try a small (child's) toothbrush with soft bristles. It might sound odd, but I assure you that having used one for several years now, it is better and more effective!

Ask the nurse about sponges on sticks that can be used to clean the patient's mouth if they cannot clean their teeth. These can also be used to moisten their mouth with water. Don't use glycerine – it dries the mouth and lips.

If the patient is very poorly, a few drops of water dripped into the mouth from a syringe will help prevent dryness and discomfort.

Explore

If the patient is sensitive about drinking from a bottle of water while in public, experiment with more discreet containers. Juice bottles with an integral folding straw, like the type sold by Lakeland Plastics, are small and easy to use.

A refillable perfume atomiser is even smaller and quickly delivers moist relief with minimal intake of fluid.

Artificial saliva sprays are available too. Ask the doctor about these. Various flavoured and unflavoured formulations are available.

More Information

Patients with a dry mouth find that some foods can be harder to eat and even painful.

Gravies are a useful way of moistening and softening food.

All forms of alcohol, including wines (red wine in particular), dry one's mouth even more than usual. Cider is often quoted as a useful agent for cleaning a dirty mouth. It is excellent at removing debris, but it is very acidic and potentially damaging to the teeth.

Avoid sugary fizzy drinks. The reason for avoiding the sugary variety is obvious – the risk of tooth decay. The sugar-free drinks also increase the risk of decay because the carbon dioxide added to make the drink fizzy also makes it acidic.

The traditional advice to 'suck boiled sweets to stimulate saliva' is a waste of time if one's salivary glands don't work properly. It's likely that they'll just rot their teeth and give themselves painful cuts to the tongue! Sugar-free chewing gum might be more suitable, but some sugar-free sweets are very acidic.

Chapter 27

The patient's mouth is sore

The doctor says

Once again, the dentist has had her say too!

Anything that makes eating or swallowing difficult for the patient deserves prompt attention. If the patient is not able to look after their own mouth care, it is essential that you check their mouth daily. They may complain of pain before any visible evidence of infection can be detected. So, don't be afraid to ask for advice and try to nip any problems 'in the bud'.

It is advisable for the patient to see the dentist or hygienist before starting treatment, if possible. If this can be done it means that any existing problems can be treated. If this is not feasible, the patient should see the dentist as soon as possible after starting treatment.

Think

A sore mouth can have many causes. Tick the problems that apply to the patient (if any of them do).

☐	Is the patient anaemic?
☐	Is the patient on antibiotic treatment? This increases the risk of thrush infection.
☐	Is the patient suffering from a dry mouth? (*See* Chapter 26.)
☐	Does the patient have any infection or ulcers in their mouth?
☐	Is the patient having chemotherapy? This may cause a sore mouth or lips, but does not always do so.
☐	Is the patient taking any other prescribed drugs?
☐	Do the patient's dentures fit badly because their gums have shrunk?
☐	Has the patient had herpes ('cold sores') following chemotherapy?
☐	Has the patient had recent or previous radiotherapy to their head or neck?

Ask

If the patient has had antibiotic treatment recently and developed a sore mouth following the antibiotic, ask the doctor or dentist for treatment for this. It could be thrush infection.

If the patient has been suffering from a dry mouth and their mouth has become sore, ask for advice about the cause.

If the patient has any form of mouth infection or mouth ulcers, report these and get treatment.

Patients receiving chemotherapy may be given treatment to prevent fungal infections, which should stop them developing thrush in their mouths. If thrush infection starts after finishing the treatment they were given, ask for advice.

If the patient's dentures fit badly they should see the dentist. A gain or loss of about 6 kilos (a stone) in weight can result in dentures not fitting as well as they should.

Patients who have had herpes simplex ('cold sores') following chemotherapy find that this infection can be quite persistent because their immune system may be suppressed by the treatment. If the infection persists or recurs, let the doctor know. It will not clear up by itself.

If the patient is suffering from a cancer of the mouth or tongue, they should report any pain promptly, especially if it has changed in any way.

Note

Patients who are having several treatments with chemotherapy at regular intervals may experience the same problems each time. Make a note of the symptoms the patient had and what treatments helped. Seek advice early if you suspect that the same problem is going to happen again.

Here are a few other things that might happen.

Patients may lose their appetite. Look at Chapter 12 'The patient has a very poor appetite' for some ideas that might help you.

Make a note of how the patient prefers their food. For example, think about:

- **temperature**: was cooler food easier for the patient to eat?
- **taste**: did the patient prefer foods that were more bland than usual?
- **texture**: did the patient find food easier to eat if it had been blended or minced?
- **moistness**: does it help to add gravy or a sauce?

Commercial dietary supplements such as Complan or Build-up might be easier to manage in the short term, but should not be used to replace the patient's normal diet for any longer than necessary.

Do ✓

Encourage excellent oral hygiene. Advise the patient to use a soft, small-headed toothbrush (e.g. a child's brush) and use a fluoride mouthwash or a fluoride gel at night. Some mouthwashes can sting, so try to find one that does not contain alcohol (e.g. Fluorigard made by Oral-B).

A home-made mouthwash with one teaspoon of sodium bicarbonate to one pint of water is soothing and helps clear the debris that collects in the mouth. The patient can use it several times a day, but should not swallow it.

Encourage the patient to tell the dentist what's been happening to them and show them all medications they are taking. Sometimes drugs can affect the mouth and gums, so the dentist needs to know all the facts in order to give you the best advice.

If patients gain or lose more than about a stone in weight, their mouths can also change shape, and their dentures might need to be adjusted to ensure a better fit. If there are problems getting the patient to the surgery, ask about a home visit from the dentist.

Explore

If you have financial difficulty and need a food blender to liquidise the patient's meals, speak to the doctor or social worker – you might qualify for a grant.

You might wish to contact the Macmillan Cancer Information Line for advice about grants and other forms of support. The telephone number is 0845 601 6161.

More Information

Mouth infections are more common in patients who are unwell. When you are tired, good oral hygiene is more difficult. Dentures and toothbrushes are notorious for harbouring infection! Bacteria just love bits of food lodged around the bristles of a toothbrush and the bathroom is usually warm and moist.

The patient's dentures should be brushed thoroughly – not just soaked. Toothbrushes must be replaced after the patient has had any mouth infection otherwise there is the risk of re-infecting themselves from a contaminated toothbrush. A simple way of reducing the risk of recurring infection is to sterilise toothbrushes etc. in 'Milton' or baby sterilising tablets made up to the strength recommended by the manufacturer. Steam sterilisers might deform the brush, so they are less practical in this situation.

Practical tips for dealing with a dry or sore mouth

- **Artificial saliva**: several artificial saliva aerosol sprays, in different flavours, are available on prescription from the doctor.
- **Chilled fruit**: chilled fruit jellies, ice lollipops or chilled slivers of pineapple to suck (discard the residue). Tinned pineapple is easier than fresh, but make sure you buy it in natural fruit juices, not syrup. Fresh pineapple can be painful on the tongue.
- **A dirty and sticky mouth** is common in the mornings. Try sodium bicarbonate mouthwashes (use 1 teaspoon in a pint of water and do not swallow the mouthwash) or try sucking pieces of tinned pineapple. Pineapple is acidic, so offer a drink afterwards to protect the patient's teeth.
- **When driving**, the patient could try drinking from a child's juice bottle or a sports training bottle with an integral straw. Keep it conveniently at hand in a holder for canned drinks hung on the door.

- **Good dental hygiene** is not so easy to keep up when one's mouth is sore. Try a soft toothbrush to minimise trauma and ask the dentist about mouthwashes to reduce inflammation or infection.
- **Ice**: a jug of iced water or a dish of crushed ice (with a spoon) is very refreshing. Ice lasts longer than water.
- **Ice cubes** can be made from any juice or sparkling water and added to water to sip. It makes tap water a bit more interesting!
- **Infection** is more common in a dry mouth because one of the functions of saliva is to act as an antiseptic. Dentures can cause minor injury to the mouth. This gives an excellent opportunity for infections to start.
- **Juices**: fresh orange, lemon or grapefruit juices are refreshing, but as these may hurt the patient's mouth, experiment first and make a note of what they liked best.
- **Mouth sprays**: a small hand-held aerosol spray filled with water or a juice of the patient's choice can be refreshing and quite inconspicuous to use.
- **Sparkling water**: tonic or soda water is refreshing. These can be made into home-made lollipops. Look for the lollipop moulds that allow melted ice to be sucked from the bottom of the mould (e.g. Lakeland Plastics).
- **Sugar-free chewing gum** can help stimulate saliva.

Chapter 28

The patient seems to be in pain

The doctor says

About two thirds of cancer patients experience pain at some time during their illness. That means that about one third of cancer patients might not suffer significant pain. Of those who do have pain, it is sometimes not well controlled. This may be due to a number of factors, including the fact that some cancer pains are very hard to control, but sometimes it is because the doctor and nurse are not told about the pain.

If you think the patient is suffering pain and not saying so, you face a difficult situation. Let's think about what you might be able to do to help.

Think

Why do you think the patient is in pain? Make a note of your reasons. Here are a few to get you started. Tick any that seem to apply and add any more that are relevant.

☐	The patient seems to be uncomfortable while sitting in a chair or lying in bed.
☐	The patient suddenly cries out as if in pain at different times.
☐	The patient cries out or groans when they move.
☐	The patient does not want to be disturbed or bothered.
☐	The patient is sleeping badly.
☐	The patient's mood has changed and they seem to be 'down' and depressed.

Ask

It's perfectly reasonable for you to ask if the patient is in pain. You must remember that you should respect their wishes if they do not want the nurse or doctor to be told about the pain. It is also quite OK for you to explore why they don't want the pain to be treated. Do remember that the patient has the right to choose to refuse any medical intervention and you can't force them to accept any help they don't want.

You might wish to ask about these possible 'reasons'. There are quite a few, so this may take a few conversations to achieve! Tick the reasons for choosing to suffer pain as they are discussed. I have included some comments below each of the reasons for refusing pain relief that you might encounter.

☐ Painkillers only mask the pain: they don't deal with the cause.
This may be true, but why suffer? If the cause can be eradicated, so much the better.

☐ Patients get addicted to strong painkillers like morphine.
When drugs like morphine are correctly prescribed, patients do not become addicted.

☐ Cancer is a painful illness – it's a fact of life.
Only two thirds of cancer patients experience pain and it can usually be controlled.

☐ A 'good patient' does not complain about pain.
No patient is expected to suffer in silence. No patient is expected to suffer at all if their pain or other symptoms can be resolved.

☐ Pain can be character-building.
Pain is more likely to be debilitating!

☐ Having pain means that my cancer is getting worse.
This is not necessarily true. There are many things that cause pain, including infections, and sometimes the pain is the result of the treatment, e.g. an operation, not the cancer.

☐ I'd prefer the pain to the side effects of the painkillers.
The side effects usually only last a few days and then settle. The pain will probably be much more persistent.

☐ It's better to save the painkillers until they are really needed.
If the patient has pain now, they need pain relief now.

☐ If I use the painkillers now, there'll be nothing strong enough for when the pain gets worse.
This commonly held belief is a complete myth. There is no 'maximum dose' of drugs like morphine. The dose required is the dose that relieves the pain.

☐ I'd rather focus on the other problems I have in case talking about my pain distracts the doctor from dealing with those issues.
The outcome of this approach is simply to distract the doctor from dealing with an important problem – the patient's pain. Encourage the patient to make a list of all the issues needing to be discussed with the doctor.

Some of these 'reasons' for refusing pain relief might sound a bit bizarre, but let me assure you, they are all relatively commonly stated concerns!

Note

Make a note of anything you feel you need to ask the nurse or doctor about with respect to the patient's pain.

Always remember that you must ask their permission to do this and that the doctor or nurse cannot discuss the patient's illness or treatment with you unless they have the permission of the patient to do so. To avoid any misunderstanding or the impression that you are holding some kind of secret discussions, I would suggest that you ask any questions or raise concerns openly in the presence of the patient.

If the patient cannot speak, make a note of what seems to cause pain – e.g. being moved or turned in bed. If they seem to be sore when touched, make a note of where they seem to have pain. There are body diagrams for you to use in Appendix 2.

Do

Encourage the patient to discuss any concerns they have about painkillers, etc.

Explore

Complementary therapies sometimes help. Acupuncture has helped some people with cancer pain. You might wish to explore the availability of complementary therapies in your area, but remember they might not be available on the NHS. Can the patient afford the fees? Can you be responsible for transporting the patient to a clinic that is not local? Ambulance or hospital transport is not provided for non-NHS clinic appointments.

More Information

Other therapies, including hypnosis and imagery, can help reduce awareness of pain. These techniques must be taught by a trained practitioner and are not available in every area. It is always worth trying simple measures such as relaxing music, television or reading a light story or magazine to distract attention. These have no effect on the severity of the pain, but can help the patient focus on something more pleasant.

Chapter 29

The patient needs practical care

The doctor says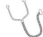

It is easy to assume that everyone is able and willing to be involved in the practical care of a relative, but it's not always the case. Even husbands and wives can have 'boundaries' about how much they can do for each other and both the patient and you have the right to express your concerns and reservations.

You and the patient must agree about how much time you have, what you are able to do and what level of intimate care you are expected and are able to give.

If you have other commitments, these should be made clear so that a suitable balance can be achieved between what you can do and when it is appropriate to ask for help from others.

Think

- How much time can you offer?
- Do you feel able to cope with most aspects of caring for the patient? If there are things that you are especially good at or things that you do not feel able to do, make a note of these in the 'Note' section below.
- Will the patient be happy for you to be responsible for their more intimate care?
- Are you happy to wash, dress and assist with bathing, etc.? You and the patient are allowed to set 'privacy boundaries'. There is no set formula for what you are expected to be able to do.
- Who else is available to give you a break? After all, you need time to relax and 'switch off' too!

Ask

Ask the patient about your involvement in their practical care. They must be agreeable for you to get to know quite a lot about their illness, their treatment and their daily needs if you are to offer the best care. If they have reservations about you being involved, discuss these early on so that appropriate arrangements can be made.

Note

Make a list of the areas where you feel confident to offer your input and a list of the things that you do not feel able to do, or those roles that the patient prefers to be taken on by someone else.

Keep a note of the names and contact numbers of the people who can offer the input and necessary care that you are not able to give for any reason.

Do   ☑

Here it is probably easiest to give a few brief suggestions about a range of practical issues. These are listed alphabetically to make them easier to find.

Bathing

Having a bath is one area where accidents can happen to both you and the patient. Many professional nurses will not attempt to lift a patient in or out of the bath without a hoist. Do not risk an injury to yourself or the patient.

If the patient is reasonably fit, grab rails, a shower seat or a bath seat may all help. If your DIY skills are not up to fitting grab rails, ask for a professional to do it for you. Ask the nurse or doctor about the possibility of borrowing bath or shower seats before going to the expense of buying your own. The occupational therapist may wish to visit and assess what is most suitable for the patient. Try a plastic garden chair in the shower in the short term.

Drinking enough

Keeping up a reasonable fluid intake when feeling unwell and possibly sick can be difficult. Try offering new flavours, including the 'isotonic' drinks suggested for use in sporting events. These are easily obtained in supermarkets and are absorbed easily and quickly. Generally speaking, fizzy drinks are less well tolerated. Cold drinks or even pieces of ice to suck are sometimes better tolerated than hot beverages. Experiment with herbal teas and even soups. Always keep a fresh drink readily available and encourage small frequent sips rather than infrequent large volumes.

Hickman lines

The care of a Hickman or PICC line is best left to the nurse. Report any unusual redness or soreness without delay – it could indicate infection.

Laundry

It is possible that the amount of laundry you need to do will dramatically increase as a result of incontinence, a weeping wound or a leaking fistula (*see* Chapter 22).

If the patient has incontinence and must get to the toilet in a hurry, the problem can be made easier by use of elasticated trousers such as jogging suits. A bottle or commode may be a useful option.

Incontinence pads can be supplied by the nurse. Store used pads in black bin liners to reduce odour and ask about whether there is a collection service for their disposal.

In spite of all these measures, extra laundry may still be a regular part of your responsibilities. You might be able to get a grant for a washing machine or tumble drier (*see* Chapter 6). If the amount of laundry you need to do daily is a problem, ask the nurse or social worker about the availability of laundry services in your area.

Meals

If you are not available to cook a meal for the patient, think about stocking up the freezer with ready-made meals, either home-made or ready frozen, to pop into the oven or microwave. If possible, home-made meals, of suitable size and made to a favourite recipe, are best.

Older patients might qualify for meals on wheels. Ask the social worker for advice.

See the tips at the end of Chapter 12 'The patient has a very poor appetite'.

Medications

Remembering what is to be taken and when can be quite a difficult problem, especially if you are not used to taking (or dispensing) tablets regularly. There are a number of different multi-section tablet boxes available to remind you what is to be taken at different times of day. Some of these can be filled once a week, which is very useful if the patient can look after their own medications.

The thing you must do is give the patient their medications exactly as prescribed. You must be aware of the names of all the medicines and tablets, what they are for and when and how they are to be taken. Sometimes extra medications are prescribed, to be taken 'as required', for example for pain that occurs in spite of the regular doses of painkillers. You need to know what to give, how much to give and how many doses can be given in 24 hours. You need to know when to call the doctor or nurse if the medications are not working as they should.

To help you give the various medicines at the correct times, a kitchen timer can be set to remind you when the next doses are due. This allows you to get on with other things until the buzzer sounds. You can also buy tablet boxes with built-in alarms!

If you have difficulty remembering what was given and when, or simply want to let someone else 'take over' and let them see what has been given, then simple home-made charts like those in Appendix 3 can help. I used charts like these when I was taking tablets several times a day. As they say, 'It worked for me', but they can only work if everyone, including the patient if they take their own medicines sometimes, uses them properly!

Sometimes patients become reluctant to take tablets and medicines. This can be for a variety of reasons. Here are some of the commoner problems and suggestions for how you can help.

- There are too many medicines and it's hard to remember what to take and when.
  Try a multiple dose box, and lists of what is to be given/has been given. See Appendix 3.
- The medication has unpleasant side effects.
  Speak to the doctor or nurse – an alternative that suits better may be available.

- The medication has a bitter or unpleasant taste.
  Ask the patient to suck an ice cube immediately before taking the medicine. This can help by numbing the taste buds and making them less sensitive.
- The patient does not believe the medications are really necessary.
  This suggests that they might be denying their illness. Denial is a basic defence mechanism which we all use to protect ourselves from unpleasant or threatening situations. Try discussing the reasons why they are necessary: if you face serious resistance, speak to the nurse or doctor.
- The patient is confused and forgetful.
  Try a multiple dose box, and lists of what is to be given/has been given. If this fails, you might have to accept responsibility for giving the medications at the appropriate times.
- The medicine is to prevent symptoms or side effects and the patient thinks they are not necessary because they have no symptoms.
  This is the proof that the medication is working! Try and explain that this is why they are symptom-free and that stopping the medicine will result in them suffering. If you fail, ask the nurse or doctor for advice.

After a visit to the hospital or admission to hospital, it is usual to be given about three days' supply of medications and a letter to the doctor. This is not a prescription, but it will list the medications to be taken. Take into account the time it takes for the doctor to process the prescription and local half-day closing or public holidays that might affect the availability of the chemist to dispense the medicines.

Mobility

Getting around can be difficult for seriously ill patients, either because they are short of breath (*see* Chapter 13) or simply because they are weak and tired (*see* Chapter 34). Think about the simple things that can help them – a raised toilet seat, or raising the bed or chair a couple of inches, which can reduce the amount of work required in getting up. Do not use bricks to raise chairs or a bed because these can slip and cause injury. Commercially made and very safe bed- and chair-raisers are available, as are raised toilet seats. Ask the occupational therapist or doctor whether these are available to borrow.

In the longer term, if getting up and down stairs to go to the bathroom is getting too much, consider moving the bed downstairs, if the bathroom is on that level, or bring a chair up to the bedroom so that the patient can have a change of position.

Alternatively, a commode downstairs might save a few extra journeys.

Some of these ideas might not be the most desirable changes to have to make, but at least the patient can remain involved with their family and not be isolated as well as ill.

Night-time care

It is not easy to be 'on call' 24 hours a day, seven days a week. If the patient needs you during the night, you might be able to get some extra help. Marie Curie nurses can sometimes stay with the patient if you are not able to do so and sometimes night sitters can offer you a 'night off'. These services are in heavy demand and help might not be available as often as you would like, but your need will be fairly assessed and you will be given the help available. Ask the district nurse, Macmillan nurse or doctor about the support available in your area.

If the patient qualifies for Attendance Allowance, you might be able to use some of this extra money to pay for a private nurse or non-qualified person to stay on a couple of nights a week and give you some time off. Carefully assess the needs of the patient before choosing a suitably qualified carer to be there in your absence.

Citizens Advice Bureaux offer independent advice on benefits. Other useful contact numbers are included in Appendix 4, 'Useful organisations'.

Skin care

The patient's skin could be at risk for several reasons. These can categorised in four basic areas:

- friction
- moisture
- pressure
- swelling (e.g. lymphoedema).

A word of warning at this point – do not use ring-shaped cushions. They actually increase the pressure on the skin and can do more harm than good.

Friction damage can occur during movement, either from vulnerable skin rubbing on the sheets or from shearing and friction when being moved in the bed. If vulnerable areas like elbows and heels are showing signs of becoming red and sore, try to protect these with longer sleeves, socks or lambswool skin protectors which can often be obtained from the community nurses or can be purchased through several larger chemists networks, e.g. Boots and Lloyds. Further details are included in Appendix 4.

Moist skin, whether from excessive sweating, incontinence or a persistently leaking wound, is more vulnerable to infection and breakdown. Speak to the nurse about how to absorb or reduce excess moisture and minimize the risk of skin damage.

On the other hand, excessively dry skin can crack and become vulnerable. Use only a good quality non-perfumed moisturiser and use a barrier cream if the patient is incontinent.

Pressure on the skin can result from sitting or lying in one position for too long. Try to encourage regular and frequent changes of position to reduce this risk.

Any swelling, but lymphoedema (*see* Chapter 25) in particular, puts the skin at risk. Lymphoedema usually affects one limb and usually results from damage to the lymph glands in the armpit or groin after surgery or radiotherapy. Look out for any minor breaks in the skin surface or leakage of fluid. Report these immediately as there is a substantial risk of infection.

Toilet problems

One of the commonest problems regarding the toilet is access. A breathless patient or one who is too weak to climb the stairs to the bathroom can end up isolated in a bedroom upstairs because that's the easiest option.

Think about the option of borrowing a commode. They can dramatically reduce the amount of effort required to get up and down stairs or even make a journey that is too long. If everything is on the one level, think about putting a chair half way between the bedroom and bathroom to 'break the journey' if the patient is breathless or gets tired very easily.

Think too about the issue of adequate privacy for using the commode. A separate room is obviously the ideal, but even a tri-fold screen, which someone reasonably competent at DIY could make, could be sufficient to hide the commode from view when visitors call.

Ask the community nurse about borrowing a commode. I guess the screen will have to be your responsibility!

Washing the patient

Regular washing or a 'freshen-up' is something every patient will appreciate. A bath may not be possible, but a shower, if the patient is fit enough, requires less effort in terms of standing and sitting. A plastic garden chair might allow the patient to sit in the shower.

If a shower is not possible, provide a basin and assist with washing, paying particular attention to any vulnerable areas of skin. Generally speaking, a non-perfumed soap or baby bathing products are usually well tolerated.

If the patient is having radiotherapy, special care of the affected area of skin is essential. Follow the instructions given by the radiotherapy department, but avoid soap and do not use talcum powder or any creams without consulting the radiotherapy staff. Talcum powder and many creams contain minute particles of metal which can cause the radiotherapy beam to be deflected away from the intended area.

Wound care

Generally speaking, this is the forte of the nurse. Ask for advice and do exactly as you are advised.

Explore

Don't try to undertake any form of care that you are not competent to give. Always ask for advice or a demonstration of what you are trying to do. The nurse and doctor are your first contacts and the occupational therapist can advise about aids and appliances. The social worker will advise about finances and grants. Cancer patients who need equipment such as washing machines to help cope with an increased amount of laundry might be able to get a grant from Macmillan Cancer Relief. *See* Chapter 6 for further details.

More Information

Several support agencies exist to offer help and support to carers. Details of some of these are given in Appendix 4.

Chapter 30

The patient is having radiotherapy

The doctor says

It's over 100 years since the accidental discovery of 'radium' and the discovery of 'X-rays'. The early scientists were intrigued by how photographic paper, stored carefully in the dark, became 'fogged'. It was not long before the invisible radiation was associated with radium and soon it was discovered that this invisible ray left a mark on photographic paper and could be used to make pictures of the bones in one's hands.

The early pioneers of radium and X-rays all suffered serious skin burns and illness as a result of the excessive exposure to the effects of these dangerous rays. In spite of this, it was popular in the 1920s to drink irradiated water for the good of one's health!

The sufferings of the early scientists remind us that radiation can burn the skin and excessive doses of radiation can do harm as well as good.

Think

- There are several methods used today to treat patients with radiotherapy. Do you know which regime is being used? Is it one treatment daily for four or five weeks or three treatments daily for seven days?
- Are you familiar with the precautions to be taken with respect to skin care?
- Do you know what the treatment is expected to achieve? For example, is it intended to cure the cancer, dry up a wound that is leaking, relieve pressure on the spine from a tumour growing or stop bleeding from a blood vessel in the lung?
- Do you know the possible and likely effects of the treatment?
- Do you know the likely side effects of the treatment?

Ask

- If you are responsible for the daily care of the patient, ask them if they were given booklets about their treatment which you could read to be better informed about it.
- Find out about the times and frequency of the treatment sessions. Can you be available to take the patient to and from all these appointments?
- What side effects are likely? Tiredness and nausea are very common. If the treatment involves the lower bowel or bladder, some degree of urgency to find a toilet may be experienced. If you have a long journey to make to and from the treatment centre, can you plan a route that allows for a comfort break? If not, you might need to ask about suitable protection in case of 'accidents'.

Note

Skin care is very important when being treated for radiotherapy. Encourage the patient to listen very carefully to any instructions given or try to get these in writing so you know exactly what to do.

Radiotherapy to the head and neck can result in a dry or sore mouth and loss of taste. Make a note of the foods that are best tolerated.

Treatment involving the abdomen can cause sickness. Make a note of which foods are least likely to cause nausea.

Do ✓

- It might sound obvious, but you must follow all instructions about skin and general care very carefully. In general, avoid soap, talcum powder and creams unless prescribed by the radiotherapy centre.
- Do not buy or use anything not specifically approved by a staff member who is involved in the treatment. Many skin preparations contain metals and the metal causes the radiation beam to reflect away from the target area.
- Encourage the patient to take all medications prescribed for nausea or any other side effects of the treatment. They will improve reasonably quickly after the treatment is completed
- Report difficulty in eating or drinking to the staff at the radiotherapy centre or your GP. Sometimes the radiation can burn the lining of the gullet and if the patient is not able to eat and drink enough, they may need dietary supplements or specialist treatment.

Explore

If you want to find out more about the general effects of radiotherapy and learn about the different treatment regimes, look at the CancerBACUP website, where you will find lots of useful information. The address is www.cancerbacup.org.uk.

More Information 📖

One of the important things about radiotherapy is that the treatment must be given with extreme care and precision. In the introduction to this chapter, I mentioned the skin burns suffered by the early pioneers and researchers. One important aspect of modern radiotherapy is to try to minimise skin damage and maximise the radiation dose given to the tumour.

To achieve this objective, very careful planning is required. This may involve making a close-fitting plastic mask of the head or plaster casts of the body. Various marks allow the staff to position the patient in a firmly held position that can be exactly reproduced at each treatment session. This may involve minor discomfort, but it's well worth it.

The planning can take a few days, which can be frustrating, but be assured that behind the scenes there is a team of people that the patient will probably never meet, all planning the treatment to maximise the effect and minimise unwanted effects.

Chapter 31

The patient is feeling sick

The doctor says

When I was having weekly chemotherapy, I spent about three months when I felt sick every day. It is one of those symptoms that can be very difficult for you to assess in terms of how the patient feels. Only the patient knows just how bad they feel. Gradually, my confidence grew that I could eat and not actually be sick!

My nausea was slightly worse on the day *before* I was due to have my chemotherapy. Why was that? Quite simply, I believe it was anxiety about going to the hospital the next day! Yes, doctors have fears about having treatment too!

There are a number of possible causes for feeling sick (nauseated). The most effective treatment will depend on the precise cause. To determine the cause, the doctor will probably ask quite a lot of questions. The nausea might be directly due to the illness or the medications being given. Chemotherapy is a common cause of nausea, especially in the few days immediately after treatment.

When I was a medical student, I was given a tip for the exams. I was told that if I was asked about the side effects of any drug, I could always play for time by saying 'nausea' while I racked my brain for a more specific answer!

While none of us likes being sick, vomiting frequently relieves the sensation of nausea.

Possible causes of nausea include:

- worry, stress and anxiety, as I have already admitted
- anything that upsets the patient's bowel function e.g. constipation (*see* Chapter 17), indigestion or a simple tummy upset
- a build-up of chemicals in the blood due to the liver or kidneys not working as well as usual (a blood test will confirm if this is the reason)
- almost any drug can cause nausea, but strong painkillers, antibiotics and anti-cancer chemotherapy are among the common causes. Nausea associated with strong painkillers usually settles after a couple of days.

When a patient complains of nausea, this is an ideal time for the doctor to review the patient and their medications. This review could include a full examination and blood tests.

Think

Speaking from experience, patients often do not remember exactly when they started to feel sick or how bad their sickness was. It can be helpful for you to take note of what has been going on.

- When did the patient first complain of feeling sick?
- What is the pattern of their nausea? Is it intermittent or is it there all the time?
- Has this pattern changed? If it has, can you associate this change with any event?
- Is the nausea accompanied by hiccuping or retching?
- Has the patient's treatment been changed recently? Did the nausea start after that change in treatment?
- Has the patient been coughing? Sometimes bad coughing bouts result in vomiting.

Ask

Ask whether the patient's nausea is likely to be a short-term problem or more prolonged. This will help you to know which of the ideas listed under 'Do' you might need to consider.

Note

If the patient is vomiting, make a note of the times when they are sick. This can help the doctor decide the exact cause. Do any of these apply?

- The patient usually vomits, with little warning, at the end of the day.
- The patient suffers from forceful vomiting early in the day.
- The patient wakens with a headache and is sick.

Do ✓

Make sure that the patient takes any sickness medicine exactly as prescribed. Even when they feel OK, their nausea might return if they stop taking their medication prematurely, so encourage them to continue until told to stop by the doctor or nurse. It is very tempting to reduce the number of tablets one has to take daily, and sickness medication is one that we sometimes feel confident to stop taking.

There are a number of simple things you can try. Some may sound a bit strange, but they have been tried and they all worked for someone else. Tick the ones that help for future reference.

☐	Avoid giving the patient fatty/greasy foods.
☐	Offer some dry food before getting out of bed, e.g. a rich tea biscuit.
☐	After the patient has been off food for a while, resume with clear soups, etc. and build up to 'normal food' slowly.
☐	Fizzy drinks might help – ginger/mineral water/lemonade. Taking them through a straw seems to be even more effective.
☐	Offer drinks between meals rather than with meals.
☐	Sucking crystallised ginger can help car sickness.

Try and minimise exposure to the smell of food cooking (especially cabbage, from personal experience)! Here are some ideas that have been tried and tested.

- When cooking cabbage or sprouts, a small bay leaf added to the water greatly reduces the cooking smell. If you don't have any bay leaves, add a slice of bread broken into chunks. Rye bread is particularly effective.
- The smell of cauliflower cooking is reduced by adding lemon to the saucepan (traditionally half of the 'shell' of a squeezed lemon).
- The smell of fish cooking can be minimised by adding either celery stalks or leaves to the saucepan. A fishy smell on the dishes is easily removed by adding a spoonful of vinegar to the washing-up water.
- Burning a candle near the cooker can reduce cooking smells in the kitchen. Just don't leave it unattended!

Explore

You will find ideas in all sorts of places – old household recipe books, books of hints and tips, etc. Many are of the 'it worked for me' category and are harmless, even if they don't work.

I would advise caution over some of the less tried and tested ideas you might come across.

You should be aware that, no matter how 'harmless' they may appear, some complementary or herbal remedies can interfere with prescribed medications. Ask the nurse or doctor before exploring the possible use of complementary therapies (*see* Chapter 15).

These complementary therapies might help and should not affect any other treatment:

- acupuncture or acupressure
- hypnosis and imagery
- relaxation techniques.

If you are exploring these techniques on behalf of the patient, make sure that you consult appropriately qualified professionals. Some of these therapies are not readily available on the NHS and can be expensive.

More Information

When you are feeling sick, the last thing you want to do is to swallow tablets. There are several ways in which anti-sickness medicine can be given. Here are some of them:

- **injections**: either repeated as required, or via a syringe driver. When the nausea settles, you can take the tablets by mouth
- **suppositories**: inserted into the back passage
- **skin patches**: these look like a plaster for a cut, but have the medicine on a small patch and it absorbs through the skin
- **tablets that absorb** through the gums and are held in the mouth. These are not so easy to tolerate if your mouth is dry (*see* Chapter 26).

Some anti-sickness medicines can make patients sleepy. This can be helpful because if the patient feels sleepy, the sickness is likely to be less troublesome.

It's easier to assess the severity and frequency of vomiting than a report of feeling nauseated. Only the patient can tell how they feel so we, the carers, must encourage them to be open and honest in reporting how they feel.

Chapter 32

The patient's skin is at risk

The doctor says

Advancing cancer is often associated with loss of weight, weakness, reduced mobility and increasing periods of time spent in bed. Weakness can result in reduced ability to move and change position while in bed, or when sitting in a chair, and this puts the 'pressure areas' of the lower back and bottom, shoulders, heels and elbows at risk.

There are three main reasons for skin to break down. These are:

- **pressure**: weight taken on areas where 'padding' is lost due to loss of weight
- **friction**: especially if the sheets are rough or have been starched
- **moisture**: excessive sweat or incontinence. Damp skin is more prone to breaking down and becoming infected.

Frequent changes of position are essential to minimise the risk of skin becoming red and at risk. The patient needs to be *lifted* when being repositioned, not pulled up the bed or twisted round. This may require two people – can you enlist the necessary help?

It is much better to put the effort into effective skin care than allow the patient to develop a 'pressure sore'. These are hard to treat, often don't heal and can easily become infected, not to mention the pain and discomfort they cause to the patient. It doesn't take very long in one position for the skin to be put 'at risk' in a person who is not eating well, is relatively immobile and in poor health.

Think

- Why is the patient's skin at risk? Do any areas look red or broken or is he/she incontinent or sweating excessively?
- Has the patient become less mobile recently? If so, has this change followed a change in medication?
- Is the patient eating and drinking reasonably well?
- Do you feel that you are receiving the advice you need from the nurses and doctors?
- If the patient is heavy and needs assistance with moving, is a hoist or other appropriate equipment available? Do not use this type of equipment yourself without being given appropriate training.

Ask

- If you feel that a recent change in medication has caused the patient to be more drowsy or less mobile, ask if that medication can be changed or the dose modified.

- Ask for advice about how to lift the patient and how to reposition them to minimise the risk to vulnerable areas of skin.
- Ask about how to prevent damage to the skin and about the provision of any necessary aids.

Note

Regular assessment and reassessment of the skin is vital. Make a note of any areas of the skin that look red or broken. Report broken skin to the nurse or doctor before it becomes infected and develops into a pressure sore. Small breaks have a better chance of healing if treated early.

Do

- Turn the patient frequently or encourage them to change positions regularly.
- Use pillows to support the body and to separate the areas of contact – e.g. a pillow between the knees can prevent the skin from becoming red and sore.
- Move the patient by lifting (which avoids shearing forces on body tissues) – not by pushing or pulling.
- Keep the skin clean, protect it from injury and don't let it remain wet if the patient is sweating or is incontinent.
- Don't let the skin become too dry. Use a good quality moisturiser if necessary.
- Wash the skin only at normal times, unless the patient is incontinent or is sweating excessively.
- Don't use creams or cosmetics except for very dry skin. Barrier creams may be useful if the patient is incontinent or needs to be washed frequently.

If the patient is suffering from incontinence of urine or faeces (bowel content), skin care measures are even more important.

Patients with a swollen limb due to lymphoedema (*see* Chapter 25) are at even greater risk and need even more meticulous skin care.

Explore

Various aids and appliances are available that help to relieve pressure. You will find all kinds of devices advertised in magazines and on the Internet.

Choosing an appropriate pressure-relieving device is the role of the trained professional and I really do not recommend that you try to find your own way through the maze of products available.

Cushions for wheelchairs need to be of the correct size and of a type suited to the weight of the patient. Pressure-relieving mattresses come in a variety of types and it is best left to the experts to advise which type is most suited to the individual needs of the patient.

More Information

Sheepskins help keep the skin dry and help to reduce friction. They do not relieve pressure. Use of a sheepskin does not mean that the patient does not still require regular turning and skin care.

Ring cushions are popular and are frequently advertised in magazines and 'health catalogues'. They can interfere with the circulation and should not be used.

Chapter 33

The patient has difficulty swallowing

The doctor says

Difficulty in swallowing or a sensation of choking on one's food are very distressing for both the patient and the carer. Patients with cancer of the gullet who have had a tube (stent) inserted are also at risk of the tube blocking with food and they may need specialist advice to clear the blockage.

There are some things that you can do to try to resolve the problem.

Think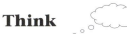

- Is the patient experiencing pain on swallowing or difficulty getting solid food down?
- Is the patient suffering from cancer of the throat or gullet (oesophagus)?
- Has the patient had a tube inserted to ease previous swallowing difficulty?

If it is available, radiotherapy to the inside of the gullet can be effective in controlling symptoms from tumours obstructing the passage of food down the gullet.

Ask

- Ask the patient whether they have been experiencing any problems with swallowing solids and if the problem has been gradually getting worse.
- Ask whether there is any difficulty swallowing liquids. (This information will help the doctor or nurse to decide the likely cause of the problem.)
- Find out if the patient has been eating stringy or pithy foods such as oranges, which can stick and form a mesh in which other food particles can become trapped.
- Is the difficulty in swallowing due to discomfort alone or because the food will not go down?
- Has the patient got a dry or sore mouth (*see* Chapters 26 and 27)?
- Are there any other problems, e.g. difficulties with speech?
- If the problem is an ongoing one, ask about soft or liquid diets and whether the patient should see a dietician.

Note

Make a note of any recent changes to the patient's diet in case there is a food that is sticking and causing a blockage. In general terms, pithy or stringy fruits and pieces of meat which have not been chewed enough or are too big are common culprits.

Tubes (stents) inserted to help swallowing in cases of cancer of the oesophagus (gullet) most commonly become blocked by either of these two foods.

If the patient has recently been treated for any infection of the mouth or throat, make a note of this and mention it to the nurse or doctor. Sometimes infection can recur and cause problems with swallowing – usually due to discomfort rather than a blockage.

Do

- Encourage the patient to sit as upright as possible when eating and drinking. This helps food to go down more easily.
- Make sure that food is soft and moist as this is easiest to swallow.
- Avoid bread and stringy foods. Make sure meat is cut very fine or minced.
- If necessary, mince all foods as these slip down more easily.
- Encourage the habit of drinking during the meal to wash food down and minimise the risk of food sticking.
- If the patient has a tube inserted, it is essential that food is soft, free from any lumps and sufficiently moist. Encourage the patient to have a fizzy drink after the meal to dislodge any small particles of food and reduce the risk of blockage.
- Check whether tablets can be prescribed as liquid preparations. If not, ask the doctor, nurse or pharmacist about whether they can be crushed. Do not crush tablets without asking first – some drugs are designed to be released slowly from the tablet (e.g. MST and MXL) and crushing these will result in the patient receiving a much larger amount of the drug and could result in overdosing.

If the problem persists despite these measures, ask the doctor for advice.

Explore

Ask about a 'Doidy cup' at the chemist's or in a shop specialising in the needs of less able-bodied people. A Doidy cup has slanted sides and is easier for the patient to drink from. If you have problems obtaining a Doidy cup, speak to the occupational therapist, who may be able to help you obtain one.

If you can't find a Doidy cup, you could try making a 'cutaway cup' from a polystyrene picnic cup (the type that prevents you burning your fingers). Using sharp scissors or a craft knife, cut away a portion of the cup – the dark part in the illustration. This allows the patient to drink without tilting their head and allows room for their nose. It can make swallowing much easier.

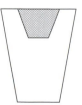

Figure 33.1 The home-made 'cutaway cup'.

More Information 📖

If the problem with swallowing is persistent or the cancer is growing and causing obstruction to the oesophagus, there are other options available, which the doctor will discuss with the patient. These include:

- an operation to relieve the blockage
- insertion of a tube or stent to prevent the tumour narrowing the gullet any further
- chemotherapy or radiotherapy as appropriate
- laser treatment to reduce the tumour size
- a 'PEG' tube (a tube inserted through the abdomen directly into the stomach allowing feeding but avoiding the need to swallow).

Obviously none of these procedures offer a cure and are only intended to provide relief of a distressing symptom.

If it becomes difficult even to swallow saliva, the doctor or nurse may suggest a treatment that will reduce the amount of saliva produced. This can result in a dry mouth (*see* Chapter 26).

Chapter 34

The patient is weak

The doctor says

We all get tired when we have cancer and are having chemotherapy and radio-therapy. I am not talking about simple tiredness in this chapter but about weakness when the patient finds it increasingly difficult to carry out their usual daily activities.

As disease advances, this can become quite a distressing problem. Gradually increasing weakness can become bad enough for patients to need to spend most of their time in bed or sitting in a chair, but a sudden onset of weakness can occasionally result in them becoming completely immobile if not reported and dealt with quickly.

Think

- Has the patient's weakness come on slowly and gradually or suddenly?
- Has the patient had more pain recently? Are they less active because of pain?
- If the patient admits to any back pain, loss of feeling in their feet or legs, or any difficulty passing urine, report these *immediately* to the doctor.
- Has the patient had a fall recently and been weak since that event?
- Has the patient been feeling sad or depressed (*see* Chapter 18)?
- Has the patient's treatment been changed recently?
- Has the patient's blood been checked recently? They could be anaemic.

Ask

- If the patient's weakness has come on *suddenly*, speak to the doctor *urgently*. Delays in treatment could result in permanent weakness or paralysis in some cases.
- If the patient's pain has increased, speak to the nurse or doctor and have their pain assessed and treatment reviewed.
- If the patient has had a fall, report this to the doctor. They might have broken a bone.
- If the patient's treatment was changed recently and their weakness came on since that change, ask the doctor or nurse if these events could be related.
- If the patient is feeling sad or depressed, speak to the nurse or doctor.
- Ask about a blood test to exclude anaemia if this has not been done for some time.

Note

Make a note of when the patient first became weak, any changes that were made in their treatment just before the weakness started and any other significant event.

Do

Advise the patient to try to avoid standing. A chair in the shower or bathroom may help. If you don't have a shower seat, a plastic garden chair will do. Standing showering, with the warm steamy air, can make patients feel quite light-headed. They may wish to sit down after a shower too.

If the patient is offered physiotherapy, hydrotherapy (a bit like a swimming pool) or exercises, make every effort you can to help them attend for these therapies. Initially it may be very tiring for them, but the exercise will help them build up the strength in their muscles and prevent or delay the onset of further weakness.

Encourage the patient to take their medications as prescribed and not to stop any tablets or medicines unless told to do so by the nurse or doctor.

Explore

A wheelchair can be very valuable in making it possible for the patient to get around and possibly get out in the fresh air. Wheelchairs can usually be supplied by the doctor or occupational therapist, but if there is a delay in getting a suitable wheelchair, the Red Cross might be able to lend you one. You might wish to explore this.

Equipment to lift the patient and help you with bathing and getting them into and out of bed is usually provided by the nurse or occupational therapist. The equipment should be used by trained persons. Do not attempt to buy these devices yourself.

Find out about local taxi firms that can take wheelchair passengers and inquire about reduced fares for disabled passengers on public transport. This can enable the patient to enjoy many of these activities and there are hotels that have specially designed facilities for guests with disabilities.

Ask about a disabled person's badge for the car (it can be put on your car if you are responsible for transporting the patient) to facilitate parking in designated places that allow the patient easier access to shops or other public places.

More Information

Sudden weakness or rapidly worsening weakness, especially when associated with difficulty in passing urine, can be caused by pressure on the spinal cord. This may be due to the cancer growing and causing compression of the spinal cord. This will not resolve by itself and requires **urgent** action. Report it immediately. Delays in starting treatment can result in permanent loss of function that can sometimes be prevented by early intervention.

In the first instance the doctor will probably prescribe a high dose of steroids to reduce the swelling around the tumour. This is not a permanent solution and it is likely that the patient will require urgent hospital treatment. They might need radiotherapy to shrink the tumour or even surgery to stabilise the spine and prevent further pressure and permanent loss of feeling and movement.

Hints for helping the patient who is tired and weak

Invite the patient to make a list of the activities that they find exhausting. Can you help with any of these, or even do them for the patient?

- Encourage the patient not to waste energy doing things you can do for them. They will probably resist help at first, but hopefully will soon recognise this as an important part of your role as their carer.
- Encourage the patient to use their energy for things they want, and need, to do most.
- Help the patient to plan their day. Is there a time when they feel at their best? This might be the best time for having visitors and doing things they enjoy.
- Washing and dressing are exhausting. Advise a short rest between the various stages.
- Ask the patient to make a list of the things they want to do today. Advise them to tackle the most important ones first. Sometimes, doing the things you least enjoy first gets them over and done with, allowing them to focus on a more enjoyable activity later when they are likely to be more tired. This can reduce the stress associated with weakness and constant tiredness.
- Make sure the patient doesn't try to do more than they can cope with.
- For regular journeys, e.g. to the bathroom, place a chair about halfway along. This allows for frequent rests and may allow the patient to remain independent for a little longer.
- Sitting near an open door for fresh air can be refreshing.
- Dizziness is common, especially on rising from bed. Advise the patient to get up in three stages:
  - sit on the bed for 30 seconds
  - stand up for 30 seconds
  - move off slowly.
- Reading, music, prayer and meditation can all help people relax and sleep at night. The routine use of sleeping tablets is seldom the best answer.

The following symptoms should be reported to the doctor:

- severe or worsening dizziness
- falls, especially if there is injury or unconsciousness.
- breathlessness – if a new symptom or worse than usual
- the patient cannot be roused
- the patient has refused to get out of bed for several days.

Psychological, Social and Spiritual Issues

Chapter 35

The patient's cancer was in remission but has recurred

The doctor says

We are always hopeful that treatment for cancer will result in a cure but, realistically, we know that this is not always the case. Sometimes the treatment achieves a 'remission' of disease that can last for some time. What exactly is 'remission'?

Stedman's medical dictionary defines remission as an 'abatement or lessening in severity of the symptoms of a disease'. In other words, there can be quite a period when there are no symptoms present and the disease seems to have disappeared. Gradually we relax and begin to think we might be cured. It is always disappointing when something happens to make us aware that the cancer may once again be active.

'Cure', in respect of cancer, is usually taken to mean that disease has permanently disappeared and never recurs. As a doctor, I was always wary of using the word 'cured' with my cancer patients, preferring to say that the chances of them developing further disease were no greater than those of any individual chosen at random from the general population. In other words, any of us can develop cancer. On average, one person in three will, so we are all at some risk.

Think

Being told that cancer has recurred is always very difficult, both for the patient and the carer.

Who told the patient (or you) that the cancer has recurred? Was this information given on the basis of tests and a full examination, or is it an assumption because something has happened that seems to indicate that the cancer is active again?

Ask

Mistakes and errors in diagnosis are, thankfully, fairly rare occurrences. Doctors can't afford to 'get it wrong' but there is always the temptation to ask, especially when it's something we don't want to hear.

If a doctor or senior nurse has not given the patient the news of the recurrence, they should ask for confirmation of the facts. You, as the carer, also need to know if the disease has recurred and what extra or different care the patient will require now and as the disease progresses. You might need to consider increasing your input in terms of time and the practical care needed and think about how this fits in with your work and other commitments.

Note

It is likely that a range of tests will have been done or will be arranged when a recurrence is suspected. Make a note of dates and venues and whether you need to arrange transport or take time off to take the patient yourself.

Often repeat treatment sessions are planned at this stage. Make a note of what is being planned – is it the same as the previous treatment or is it, for example, a one-off session of radiotherapy?

You probably won't be thinking very clearly if you have just been given this news, so keep your notebook handy and jot down new questions as they come to mind.

Do ✔

Hearing that one has a recurrence is devastating news. I know: I've had three recurrences of my cancer so far. Some cancers will recur and can be kept under pretty good control for some time and respond to different treatments. Others are less responsive when they recur. The only way to know is to ask the specialist.

The thing to do is to encourage the patient to accept the treatment offered and persevere with the treatment, through the unpleasant side effects and dark days ahead.

Offer all the practical and psychological support you can. It is a difficult time for the patient and for you. There is a different anxiety associated with treatment of a recurrence as one is often afraid to hope for as good an outcome as 'first time around'.

Explore 🚲

There is not much to explore in this situation. Obviously it is perfectly fair to ask the doctor or specialist nurse about whether there are other treatments that can be tried if the chosen regime is not showing the responses one hoped for.

I do not recommend that one searches the Internet for untested and unproven 'cures'. My personal experience of this is that none of my patients ever achieved any benefit and many spent large amounts of money in the process.

More Information 📖

It is difficult to predict how well one will respond to treatment for a recurrence. One (very general) rule is that the longer the time between the original treatment and the need for a second treatment session, the better the probable response. This is something the patient may wish to ask about for planning the future.

Chapter 36

The patient's treatment does not appear to be working

The doctor says

I've said it before and I must say it again. It is up to the patient to decide how much you are told about their illness and the treatment they are receiving. Some patients don't wish to talk about their problems, their fears, hopes and expectations. There may be many reasons for this and it's not uncommon for relatives and friends to have different expectations from those of the patient.

If you do choose to ask the patient what the treatment was meant to achieve, be prepared for them to exercise their right to privacy. Even husbands and wives don't always share these details. I have cared for patients who were married for many years and I was strictly forbidden to tell the spouse about the patient's illness or the intended or likely outcomes of treatment.

Think

- What do you believe to be the likely outcome of the treatment?
- Why do you think it is not working?
- Are there signs that the disease is recurring?
- Is the patient experiencing more discomfort, fatigue or weakness?

In answering these questions, it might help for you to consider:

- previous conversations with the patient
- the patient's treatment to date and any changes that have been made
- the current status of the patient's disease.

If the patient does not appear to share your view that the treatment is not working, it is also important to consider whether the patient may be in denial of the progression of illness and/or of its likely outcome. You need to deal very sensitively with this issue.

Ask

If appropriate, you may wish to ask the patient:

- How they think their treatment is working?
- What were the patient's expectations of treatments? Are these being fulfilled?
- How does this affect the patient's view of his or her future?

Note

Make a note of any changes that you see in the patient's condition. If you think they are in pain, are being sick, are tired or are suffering other symptoms which appear to be getting worse, make a note and discuss these with the patient.

If the patient is incapable of giving an accurate history of their symptoms, these notes may prove valuable when discussing the patient's progress with the doctor or nurse.

Do

If you are in charge of the patient's medications, make sure these are taken exactly as prescribed. If the patient looks after their own medicines, encourage them to take their drugs as directed.

Make sure that the patient attends all appointments and encourage them to report any problems or changes in how they are feeling. The doctor can only prescribe effective treatment if given an accurate history!

Explore

If you are the patient's main carer, you may wish, with their consent, to explore the different options and treatments available to them at this stage of their illness. Patients are often afraid to admit that treatment does not seem to be working as well as they hoped. This may be because:

- they are disappointed and don't want to face the facts
- they don't wish to sound critical of, or ungrateful for, the help that was given.

Staff will not see an accurate report, based on careful observation, as a criticism. They need to know when treatment is genuinely not achieving the desired outcome. On the other hand, the patient does have the right to choose not to continue with treatment and may feel that they can't cope with any more.

More Information

When treatment appears not to be working, it is tempting to explore other possible therapies and I have had patients who have bought medicines over the Internet. I must say that these never worked, but I think it is only fair to include a brief outline of the current situation in the UK regarding supply of drugs online.

The Medicines Act regulates the *supply*, not *acquisition*, of those medicines obtainable only on prescription. It is therefore legal for you to try and obtain prescription-only medicines from other sources. How easy is this and what are the problems?

To obtain a prescription-only medicine, you must first get the necessary prescription from a registered practitioner, usually a doctor, dentist or nurse, and collect the drugs from a pharmacist on production of that written prescription.

You can buy prescription-only medicines in some countries without a written prescription unless the drug is a 'controlled drug', e.g. morphine. It is not an offence for you to purchase in this way, or for you to import the drug back into the UK if it is for use by yourself or a member of your household.

You can also obtain prescription-only medicines over the Internet. UK sites will require the prescription to be given to them first, just as in the pharmacy. Similar laws apply in the USA, but there are countries that will supply without a prescription.

So, what are the problems?

First, how do you know medication what to ask for? Some websites do include medical history questionnaires but these are sometimes of such poor quality that the resulting diagnosis is incorrect and the wrong treatment is offered.

Second, some suppliers will not supply overseas customers (even though the advertising suggests that they do).

Third, some of the products may be out-of-date and poorly packaged, with inadequate or misleading instructions for use. The descriptions of some medicines have been found to be inaccurate. The products supplied can be of substandard quality, having been manufactured in laboratories with poor quality control standards.

Finally, your confidentiality is not guaranteed.

If you wish to find out more about this subject, look at the UK Medicines Healthcare Regulatory Authority website (www.mhra.gov.uk/news/news/htm# internet), where you will find more warnings about the dangers of buying medicines online.

In the USA a similar website (www.fda.gov/cder/drug/consumer/buyonline/ guide.htm) warns of the risks of pursuing this course of action.

You'll see that I don't recommend online buying and not only because there are no real safeguards for you, the consumer.

It is always difficult and disappointing for the patient and their relatives when treatment does not work. It may be a little easier to accept if discussions between the doctor and patient are open and honest and if the patient shares the information about the expected course of the disease and likely outcome of treatment with the family and other carers.

Chapter 37

Taking the patient home from hospital

The doctor says

However good they are, hospitals are not our homes and there is no bed like one's own! It has been noted repeatedly that patients with a terminal illness would much rather be at home in their last weeks or days.

Obviously we all want to do what the patient wishes and it is very hard to refuse a request for care at home. This is why it is so important that we make plans with our patients and don't make promises that we later find impossible to keep.

Think

Is it the patient or you who wants the patient to be at home? Patients often wish to come home to:

- see their home for the last time
- be with the family and feel more 'in control' – even for a very short time
- have the privacy to speak to their family and say their 'goodbyes'
- complete some unfinished (private) business
- reflect on their situation and get the illness into perspective.

Family members might wish the patient to be at home in order that they can be more involved in their care.

Before taking any action and arranging to have the patient at home, think about the practical issues.

- What is your own state of health? Are you fit for the responsibilities of 24-hour care, seven days a week?
- Who is available to help you and give you time off for rest and essential activities such as shopping?
- Can you be available at all the times when the patient might need you?
- Do your perceptions of the care you can offer match the expectations and needs of the patient?

Think about the practical issues such as access to the toilet, the patient's ability to climb stairs and ensuring that there is adequate space for any essential equipment that might be required.

Are any adaptations required before the patient comes home? For example, do you need a raised toilet seat or grab rails on walls to help the patient maintain their independence? Do you need to borrow a commode? How long does it take for these arrangements to be put in place?

Ask

Successful care at home often depends on careful planning. You might wish to ask about the following.

- What support is available in the community – e.g. nursing or personal care?
- Find out, with the patient's consent, what their needs and treatment regimes are. Is there anything you need to be taught about or find out how to do?
- If the patient is only coming home for a few days and then returning to the hospital or hospice, will they have enough medications supplied to cover their time at home or do you need to obtain these from the family doctor?
- What are the arrangements for re-admission if you can't cope, or the patient wishes to go back into hospital or their condition deteriorates? Can their bed be kept for an agreed period of time (e.g. 48 hours) to let you see how practical it is to care for the patient at home?

If possible, try and arrange for a discussion with the staff about the patient's needs in terms of their daily care. If necessary, ask for basic training in how to lift or reposition the patient or help them move from their bed to a chair.

Ask about any special needs the patient has. These could include:

- bath seats
- bed-raisers
- commode
- dietary advice
- dressing of a wound or pressure area
- handrails
- raised toilet seat
- wheelchair.

Arrangements for the supply of aids and appliances differ in different parts of the country. Check what happens in your area and how long it will take for essential equipment to be supplied or fitted. What is the cost?

Note

Make a note of the names and contact details of any of the professional carers whom you might need to contact if you experience any difficulties. Since an individual can't be on duty every day, ask about a second person who can advise you in their absence.

Do ✓

Make sure that you are aware of any appointments that have been made for the patient to have tests or follow-up assessments. Check that you can get the patient to these appointments or make suitable arrangements for transport for these essential visits. You do not want to compromise treatment by giving in to a request for care at home!

Explore

In order to offer the patient the best quality of care at home, you might need the support of professional carers and the local support services. Sometimes a pre-discharge home assessment visit can be arranged so that potential difficulties can be noted and any necessary equipment can be ordered in advance.

Sometimes the occupational therapist can visit the house to see the layout and offer you advice regarding what level of assistance or adaptations are required for best patient care.

If necessary, the Social Work Department can conduct a community care assessment.

If the patient's condition permits, arrangements may be made for attendance at a day care unit on one or more days a week. This allows the relatives to have time for other duties and activities – including a 'rest day'.

Day care centres offer a wide range of creative and social activities as well as medical input, physiotherapy, occupational therapy, hairdressing, chiropody and beauty treatments.

More Information

Being a carer, one can feel isolated but there are various agencies that can help. Here are some suggestions you might wish to consider.

Community care

Social services have a statutory responsibility under community care legislation to conduct assessments that take account of the needs of individuals and their carer. Contact your local social services area office.

District nurses

Local district nurses can provide practical nursing help with dressings, supervision of medication and other nursing roles. Ask the patient's GP for advice.

Home care teams

In some areas there are home respite teams who will provide up to 24-hour home nursing care in the last few days of life. It is unrealistic to expect a family carer to be available 24 hours a day. One should not feel guilty for accepting this kind of help if it facilitates keeping a dying relative at home in the last days of their life, thus allowing them to die at home if this was their wish.

Marie Curie

Marie Curie nurses may be available to provide night-time or 24-hour home care. The costs are usually met jointly by the Marie Curie Foundation for Patients with

Cancer and the health authority. Health authorities provide night sitter services on an intermittent basis to allow respite for carers.

Meals-on-wheels service

This service, normally provided by local authorities, delivers a hot midday meal daily to the home and may be the mainstay of the patient's diet. A nominal charge is made.

Practical help in the home

Practical aid may be provided by a home help, employed by the local authority. Referral is via the local social services department.

Private practical or nursing help

Commercial agencies in most areas will put relatives and patients in touch with domestic help, companions or nurses. The social worker can often advise of what private services are available in your area.

Spiritual support

The hospital chaplain may liaise with the patient's minister or priest. The patient may request a visit from a named minister. Most ministers will be happy to visit and offer spiritual support, even if the patient has not been a regular church attendee. *See* Chapter 38 'The patient wishes to discuss spiritual matters'.

The patient wishes to discuss spiritual matters

The doctor says

It is increasingly recognised by the nursing and medical professions that the concept of 'spirituality' is not necessarily the same as being 'religious' and goes beyond religious affiliation, seeking a meaning and purpose in life, even among those who do not believe in God.

Your definition of spirituality may not include an allegiance to any formal religion. Does the patient use the term 'spirituality' when you would refer to 'religion'? You might need to distinguish between the patient's spiritual, religious and emotional needs.

In this chapter, we will think about both the meaning of the illness and the place of religious belief in the patient's life. Because you might have a different faith from that followed by the patient, a brief summary of the commoner religions is included in the following pages.

While I was researching this book, I interviewed a number of carers and this chapter is my response to the various issues raised during those interviews. It would be impossible to cover every religion and denomination and I have included a short list of books that you might find helpful.

Think

In his poem 'The Dry Salvages'[1] TS Eliot includes the line, 'We had the experience but missed the meaning'.

The patient has had the experience of illness and both of you may also have been asking, 'What is its meaning?' Have you been searching for answers to the questions like, 'Why him/her?', 'Why now?' and so on? If you are like me, you probably have not found any answers.

Is the patient seeking spiritual support? What exactly is it that they are asking for? Is it emotional support; help with searching for a meaning to life and the illness? Is the patient afraid to die without making peace with God?

I recognise that you may have no religious affiliation or you may belong to a different faith from the Christian faith, which is my own background. Do you feel able to help? If not, who can offer advice?

The patient may be anxious about dying without making peace with God. In these circumstances, a visit from a minister should not be delayed. Most churches have the name and contact details of the minister displayed outside on a notice board so it should be relatively easy to contact a minister from the appropriate denomination.

Ask

Having found out what type of help the patient is seeking, do feel able to help or do you need to ask another person to advise you?

It should be reasonably easy to find a minister or adviser from the patient's particular faith and ask them to visit. The patient might know whom you should contact. If not, the local library, Citizens Advice Bureau or the Yellow Pages might be useful resources.

The situation in hospitals is changing and there is an increasing tendency for the patient to have to 'make the first move' with respect to a visit from a chaplain.

Some patients wish to have a non-religious contact. They should ask the staff what arrangements they have for such a visit. Some hospitals have Spiritual Care Co-ordinators who visit and assess who is the best person to help with the broader issues of 'spirituality'.

As a carer, you are also going through a stressful time and you might also find it helpful to meet with a spiritual adviser at this time.

Note

Make a note of any names and contact numbers you are given. You might not wish to pursue the matter just now, but it is always useful to have the details handy.

Do

In my experience, the relief and peace of mind experienced by patients who have spoken to someone about spiritual and religious issues has been obvious to family and staff alike.

On this basis, I would suggest that this is something that you should encourage the patient to do sooner rather than later.

Explore

A World Health Organization Expert Committee on Palliative Care stated that patients have the right to expect that their spiritual experiences will be respected and listened to with attention.

It has been noted, in various studies over several years, that patients with a strong religious belief maintain their sense of control, hope and the meaning and purpose in life.[2]

You might wish to explore these ideas further.

More Information

It is possible that the patient belongs to a different religious faith from yours and you may not be familiar with certain customs and practices that are important to them. On the following pages, I will try and outline some of the beliefs of the major religions. Space does not allow a detailed discussion, but a short list of other resources is included at the end.

Because the most commonly followed faith in Britain is Christianity, I have placed it first. The other religions are listed alphabetically. Where possible, I have quoted from the religious books relevant to the religion but in some cases it has been difficult to give easily accessible references.

References

1   Eliot TS (1963) The Dry Salvages. In: *Collected Poems 1909–1962*. Faber & Faber, London.
2   Koenig HG, Larson DB and Larson SS (2001) Religion and coping with serious medical illness. *Annals of Pharmacotherapeutics*. **35**(3): 352–9.

Christianity

Origin

Christianity began about 2000 years ago and the name refers to those who follow Jesus Christ. Christianity is unique in that the Bible teaches that Jesus was crucified and died but was resurrected to life again three days later and remains alive today in Heaven.

Books and writings

The Holy Bible (Old and New Testaments) is the basis for all the teachings of the Christian faith. Quotations used here are from the New International Version of the Bible.

There are many denominations within the Christian faith and the patient will usually prefer to see a minister from their own denomination. Most hospital chaplains will be able to offer spiritual help until the patient's preferred minister is available.

Summary of teachings

God is triune – Father, Son and Holy Spirit. Jesus Christ is the one and only Son of God.

The Bible teaches that God created man (Genesis 1:27 – 'So God created man in his own image, in the image of God he created him; male and female he created them'). Christians therefore regard human life with dignity and are opposed to any act that shortens life.

The first created man, Adam, and his wife, Eve, were placed in the Garden of Eden where Adam disobeyed God by eating forbidden fruit. As a result of Adam's disobedience (sin), everyone inherited the sinful nature. Romans 3:22–25 states, 'There is no difference, for all have sinned and fall short of the glory of God, and are justified freely by his grace through the redemption that came by Christ Jesus. God presented him as a sacrifice of atonement, through faith in his blood'.

God gave the law (the Ten Commandments) but it was obvious that no one could keep the law to God's satisfaction and a system of animal sacrifices offered on behalf of the errant sinner provided forgiveness. Later God sent His Son, Jesus, to die as the final sacrifice for our sins, thus offering forgiveness to anyone who believes.

The Gospel of John states in Chapter 3, verses 16–18: 'For God so loved the world that He gave His one and only Son, that whoever believes in Him shall not perish but have eternal life. For God did not send His Son into the world to condemn the world, but to save the world through Him. Whoever believes in Him is not condemned, but whoever does not believe stands condemned already because he has not believed in the name of God's one and only Son'.

Those who genuinely seek God's forgiveness through Jesus' death for their sins will receive it and go to Heaven, but those who do not ask God's forgiveness are destined to eternal punishment.

The Christian faith is unique in that it teaches that Jesus Christ, the one and only Son of God, died to take the punishment due to us for our sins and was then resurrected from death. Faith in His sacrificial death guarantees forgiveness and a place in Heaven. Those who do not believe remain unforgiven and will be eternally punished in Hell.

Beliefs and traditions with respect to illness

Suffering and illness are generally accepted as the result of Adam's original sin, which affects mankind universally. Many Christians therefore do not believe that God is punishing them personally, and might see the illness as an opportunity to see God at work in their lives. They might refer to the story of Job in the Old Testament, pointing out that God allowed him to be put through extreme suffering and personal loss as an example to others of his faith in God. Some Christians do regard illness and suffering as a personal punishment from God and may spend time examining what they might have done wrong.

The patient might ask for representatives of their Church to pray with them and possibly anoint them with oil as part of the Church's ministry of healing.

Terminal illness and death

There are no special preparations for death or after death. Burial and cremation are acceptable (some denominations are less accepting of cremation) and there is generally no objection to a post mortem examination of the body.

Baha'i

Origin

The Baha'i faith originated in Iran in the nineteenth century and is based on the teachings of Mizra Hussayn Ali Nuri, known to his followers as Baha'u'llah (Glory of God). He declared himself to be the manifestation of God who was to lead mankind to peace and unity and to overcome differences between the various religions that traditionally disagreed in their teaching. Baha'u'llah taught that God's plan is for a single language, currency and administrative body that will bring about universal peace and harmony.

Books and writings

The Baha'i patient may request a copy of the Baha'i prayer book and other Baha'i literature. If the patient cannot supply details of a Baha'i representative, the group may be contacted by referring to the telephone directory. If no local group is listed, the London headquarters can advise.

Summary of teachings

Baha'is teach that God is one person, not three as taught by the Bible.

Baha'is believe that Jesus Christ is not the unique Son of God, but one of many prophets. They believe that Jesus' death is not particularly significant and is not a sacrifice for our sin. Baha'is believe that the Bible is incomplete without the writings of the Baha'u'llah and that the teachings of Christianity have now been surpassed by their new revelations.

Baha'is believe that there is there is a Divine remedial judgement after death but no eternal punishment for unbelievers.

Beliefs and traditions with respect to illness

Drugs are allowed, if prescribed. Alcohol and narcotics (drugs like morphine) are forbidden, but if two doctors confirm that there is no alternative available, or that the alcohol is an essential ingredient of a medication, they can be given.

Terminal illness and death

The patient will either recite Baha'i prayers or have them read if unable to recite for oneself.

After death, the body is washed and wrapped in silk or cotton. A special ring is placed on the finger and the body placed in a coffin made of fine hard wood, stone or crystal.

Cremation is forbidden and burial should take place within one hour's journey of the place of death.

Buddhism

Note: There are several schools within Buddhism and this information is very general.

Origin

There is some uncertainty about the Buddha, but it is generally accepted that he lived between 485 and 405 BC.

Initially the Buddha lived an ascetic existence, but after a period of time, he decided that such extreme self-discipline was not satisfactory and, after a prolonged period of intense meditation, he gained insight into the Four Noble Truths, which are the core of Buddhist teachings.

Books and writings

The Buddha's teachings (dharma) were not written down during his lifetime and it was some 350 years later that Buddhist monks met to try and preserve his teachings. After initial agreement, divisions and differences emerged that have resulted in the different schools of Buddhism.

Summary of teachings

Buddhism teaches the Four Noble Truths, which are:

1 that all living things are characterised by suffering and unhappiness
2 that it is wrong desire and selfishness that cause this suffering
3 that if one removes wrong desire and selfishness then one eliminates suffering and unhappiness
4 that the way to remove wrong desire and selfishness is to adhere to the eightfold path to enlightenment.

Buddhist teaching is based on non-violence, brotherhood and hard work. Buddhists believe in reincarnation so that after death, one goes on to another life, progressing towards infinite perfection or *nirvana*. To achieve *nirvana*, total self-lessness is essential, with an absence of separateness and suffering. One must follow the eightfold path, which arises from the Four Noble Truths that lead man to enlightenment through his effort.

The patient might wish to have a small statue of the Buddha with him. They will want time for uninterrupted meditation several times during the day. The times are not fixed and the duration of meditation is a matter of personal choice.

After death, Buddhists expect to be reincarnated until they eventually reach *nirvana*.

> *When I attain this highest perfect wisdom, I will deliver all sentient beings into the eternal peace of nirvana.*
> The Buddha: quoted in the 'Diamond Sutta' or the 'Perfection of Wisdom Suttas'

Beliefs and traditions with respect to illness

Suffering is the outcome of desire. If desire had truly been extinguished and the patient had truly wanted nothing, there would have been no suffering.

The lotus flower (a water lily with its roots in the mud) is a common image in Buddhist teachings. It symbolises the belief that enlightenment (the flower) can be achieved during human suffering (the mud).

Buddhists will consent to all treatment in the palliative care context. Buddhism stresses the relief of suffering and pain in particular, but the patient may be concerned that morphine and similar drugs might cloud his mind. Buddhism strongly stresses the importance of 'mindfulness' and awareness of everything. The patient should be reassured that spiritual awareness is still possible when morphine and other strong painkillers are correctly prescribed but, if they refuse them after full explanation has been offered, their wishes must be respected. Some medications will cause unavoidable drowsiness and the wishes of the patient must be considered if these drugs are considered necessary to control symptoms such as anxiety or agitation.

Terminal illness and death

There is no special observance or rite for the dying patient, but if possible, a Buddhist monk from the same school of Buddhism should visit. The Buddhist Society in London can supply contact details. Cremation is traditional.

Chinese religions

Chinese religion is not one single belief system, but is made up of four main elements – Buddhism, Confucianism, Taoism and folk religion. The rituals of one of these may be mixed freely with the ceremonies of another.

I will briefly outline each of these.

Confucianism takes its name from Confucius, who lived between 551 and 479 BC. He encouraged worship of one's ancestors and taught that one should respect one's parents and show kindness to humanity. Confucius was not a prophet, but a travelling teacher who taught that one should practise kindness and respect.

Divination is an important part of Confucianism and texts like the *I Ching* (book of changes) are among the classic texts.

Confucianism is primarily concerned with one's moral conduct on earth, but does contain a spiritual dimension in that Confucius taught that mankind is guided by a higher authority which he called 'Heaven'. Early on it was taught that Heaven approved of harmony, which came to be seen as a balance between two forces – yin and yang. Confucians try to restore order in a world of chaos.

Taoism was founded by Lao-tzu in the sixth century BC. *Tao* means 'the way' and it is reached through meditation, chanting and physical exercise, which are believed to achieve immortality. Little is known about Lao-tzu, but the main Taoist text, *Tao-te-Ching* (Classic of the Way and its Power), is attributed to him.

Taoism teaches that through a correct balance of yin and yang one can achieve a healthy state of mind. Taoists try to appreciate, learn from and work with life's events. By following the *Tao* (the way), one can obtain long life and immortality. Immortality is interpreted in two ways – eternal life in a new body and, more symbolically, a release from the worries of everyday life.

To achieve harmony of yin and yang, a complex mixture of rituals has evolved. This includes meditation, chanting, physical exercise and natural medicines. Illness is believed to be due to an imbalance of yin and yang and the balance can be restored by use of acupuncture, which is believed to control the flow of vital energy in invisible channels in the body.

Buddhism came to China in the first century AD and influenced the development of Confucianism and Taoism. Buddhists see life's problems and difficulties as obstacles to be overcome before achieving *nirvana*.

Confucius, Lao-tzu and the Buddha all lived at around the same time and these religions may have co-existed in China.

Folk religions involve the worship of a variety of gods originating in various myths and legends.

In ancient times the farmers believed that heavenly spirits controlled the sun and rain. It became popular to believe that the spirits of deceased ancestors could possibly intervene to ensure better crops.

A number of domestic gods thus developed over the centuries. As well as appealing to these gods for good fortune, people often ask them for protection against evil.

Feng shui (wind and water) is another popular practice, involving the placing of objects in the home in a way that will be in harmony with the earth's natural forces (*ch'i*). Correct placement ensures the balance of yin and yang.

Chinese funerals are associated with elaborate ritual and ceremony in the belief that burial without proper ceremony can result in the person not finding their way to heaven but remaining as a ghost. Before the soul of the deceased can ascend to heaven, it must descend to the underworld and explain its actions during life. Good behaviour ensures a faster passage to heaven. The relatives may offer ritual sacrifices to the gods or build model cars or aeroplanes to ensure transport to heaven.

Christian Science

Origin

Christian Science started in Boston in 1879. There are no ordained clergy, but there are teachers, readers and healing practitioners. These practitioners will offer prayers for the patient and their contact details will be found in the *Christian Science Journal*.

Books and writings

The most widely read book is *Science and Health with Key to the Scriptures* by Mary Baker Eddy, published in 1875. Mrs Eddy claimed this book to be a revelation from God.

Christian Scientists might ask for a Bible, but will also wish to read *Science and Health with Key to the Scriptures* or their own daily newspaper (*Christian Science Journal*) which may be obtained from a Christian Science Reading Room which each Christian Scientist Church maintains.

Summary of teachings

God is not a person, nor is God triune. God is referred to as 'Life', 'Truth', or 'Mind'. Mankind was created perfect and never departed from that state, therefore there is no need for forgiveness. There is no eternal punishment. Because God is everything, Satan does not exist, nor does evil exist except in one's mind.

Christian Scientists dispute the reality of sickness and death. Suffering, sickness and pain are all in our mind and do not actually exist. Disease can be overcome by prayer alone. They believe that the healing miracles of Jesus recorded in the Bible are the outcome of understanding the spiritual law that is available in every age.

Christian Scientists believe that because there is no such thing as evil, there is neither a Hell nor punishment for unforgiven sin after death. Punishment for sin lasts for as long as we believe in it because it only exists in our mortal minds. A terminal illness should therefore hold no fear in this respect for the Christian Scientist.

Beliefs and traditions with respect to illness

Christian Scientists believe that, because physical illness does not exist, drug treatment is not necessary. They will accept setting of fractures and surgical treatment and some may accept analgesia for severe pain. Transplants are not normally acceptable.

Terminal illness and death

There are no special requirements as the time of death approaches, except that patients would usually wish a fellow Christian Scientist to be there to support them and their family members.

Hinduism

Origin

The word 'Hindu' originates from the word 'Sindhu', which refers to the Indus river to the northwest of India, in Pakistan. A flowing river is seen as a living symbol of ongoing life, just as the river flows into the sea and falls as rain, replenishing the rivers.

Hinduism is a mixture of religious beliefs and practices that have been practised for some 4500 years in India.

Hinduism has no single founder or prophet, but is rather a way of life that attempts to free its followers from worldly cares so that they can appreciate what is true and eternal.

How Hinduism is practised varies from region to region.

Books and writings

The earliest writings are a collection of four texts called the *Vedas*, which were written around 1000 BC. Much later on, the *Upanishads*, a collection of philosophical writings, appeared and these provide answers to life's questions about our origin and what happens when we die.

The Hindu teaching divides life into four parts:

1 **Brahmacharya**: the time of education
2 **Garhasthya**: the time of working
3 **Vanapastha**: the time of retreating and loosening worldly ties
4 **Pravrajya**: awaiting freedom through death.

The Hindu believes in a return to earth in a form that may be better or worse according to one's '*karma*'. The doctrine of 'karma' teaches that what an individual does in this world affects what happens to them in the next. Good health is regarded by some as the reward for adhering closely to the religious and moral laws.

Summary of teachings

Hinduism has thousands of gods and goddesses, although most Hindus insist that these are different manifestations of one God. Among the innumerable other gods there are three supreme gods: Brahma (the creator), Vishnu (the preserver) and Shiva (the destroyer and regenerator of life). These three form the Hindu trinity. Within Hinduism are various sects with quite different philosophies and principally worshipping one of the three supreme gods.

Worship can take place in various ways, ranging from quiet meditation to twice-daily temple visits.

Hindus believe in reincarnation, so that they are reborn into the world, with their new identity being dictated by their behaviour in the previous life. The ultimate goal is to achieve *moksha* – deliverance from time into eternity (*Brahman*) – the source and origin of creation.

Beliefs and traditions with respect to illness

Hindus have a well-defined philosophy, the *Ayurveda*, which advocates a carefully planned routine of sleep, diet, personal hygiene and physical exercise in moderation.

Some Hindus may regard their final illness as the result of some breach of this code of conduct and may feel guilt. In the western world there may be some conflict between the teachings and theories of modern medicine and the teachings of the *Ayurveda*. A Hindu priest should be asked to advise if this is causing the patient anxiety.

Washing is an important aspect of Hindu life and this includes washing the hands and rinsing the mouth before and after eating.

Fasting on a regular basis is common and this may cause concerns with respect to adequate fluid intake. Prolonged fasting may have implications for medications that should be taken after food to reduce the risk of irritation to the stomach lining. While one can advise, the final decision regarding fasting rests with the patient. Ask the doctor about alternative medications if these are available.

Personal care, including help with washing and dressing, should be done by a carer of the same sex. Hindus will not normally discuss any problems or discomfort relating to their bowel or urinary function, so constipation associated with morphine and similar painkillers may go unreported.

Terminal illness and death

Hindus believe that the body should be kept pure, as should the mind. A daily bath in running water (e.g. a shower) is the preferred method of cleansing, preferably first thing in the morning, before praying. Because Hindu teaching includes the belief that bathing renders one spiritually clean, the daily washing routine may be of particular importance to a terminally ill Hindu patient.

Most Hindus regard death as of little significance because they believe they will be at one with God in their life after death.

As death approaches, the Hindu patient will be helped by the presence of a priest (*pandit*) who can help with personal acts of worship and preparation for death, which is usually accepted philosophically, in keeping with Hindu teachings.

After death, the body may be placed on the floor (customs vary) and incense may be burned. There is no restriction on who handles the body, but post mortem examinations are strongly resisted. Cremation is the normal practice and the ashes are usually scattered over water in a river or lake. Water from the River Ganges may be brought to the funeral and in some cases the family may wish to consult with the funeral director for transportation of the body to be cremated by the River Ganges.

Humanism

Origin

Humanism is not a religion, but is included here in case you need to know more about the patient's humanist beliefs.

Humanism arose, as a movement, in the fourteenth century in Italy. Humanism was the essence of the Renaissance and involved a revival of the study of the works of the Latin and Greek philosophers, searching for what they actually meant without a specifically Christian interpretation of their writings.

Protagoras (*c* 450 BC) wrote, 'Man is the measure of all things. As for the gods, I do not know whether they exist or not. Life is too short for such difficult enquiries'.

Epicures (342–270 BC) summed up the views that were becoming accepted by a small, but growing, minority when he wrote, 'Become accustomed to the belief that death is nothing to us. For all good and evil consist in sensation, but death is the deprivation of sensation and therefore a right understanding that death is nothing makes life enjoyable'.

Humanism became a point of view asserting human dignity and values and expressing a confidence in the ability of humanity to exert control over nature and to shape society according to the needs of the people.

Modern humanism is defined as 'a philosophy that puts the emphasis on humans solving the problems of life without the dogmatic authority of secular or religious institutions'.

Summary of teachings

Humanists were tolerant of all religious viewpoints, regarding the diversity of denominations and religions as differing ways of expressing one truth. The Church was not so tolerant of this viewpoint, since it challenged the teachings of the Bible, and centuries of conflict followed. By the seventeenth and eighteenth centuries, an intellectual movement called 'the Enlightenment' had been formed. It had its roots firmly in humanism.

The Enlightenment movement had the aim of understanding the natural world and humankind's place in it solely on the basis of reason and without turning to religious belief. Most Enlightenment thinkers did not reject religion completely, but accepted the existence of God and a hereafter, while rejecting the Christian theology of creation, sin and divine damnation.

Modern humanism also embraces the following teachings:

- Rational thought and responsible behaviour will enhance quality of life on earth.
- Humans exist along with other life forms and nature is indifferent to our individual existence.
- The meaning and purpose of life must be found in living, not dying.
- Moral values are not divinely revealed, nor are they the special property of any religious tradition. They must be found by humans by use of natural reasoning and our belief in what is right or wrong must be constantly subjected to the deepest reflection in light of our evolving understanding of our nature and our world.
- Humanists have faith in the human capacity to choose good over evil, but without the expectation of any reward in another life.

Beliefs and traditions with respect to illness

In terms of palliative care and the issues concerning advance directives (living wills), Dr James Fletcher, who was voted Humanist of the Year in 1974, said, 'We should drop the sanctity-of-life ethic and embrace a quality-of-life ethic'.

Humanists will accept treatment, but may ask for consideration of an advance directive (living will). Depending on the content and where you live, these documents may contain requests that cannot be carried out legally by the medical or nursing professions. Advance directives are further discussed in Chapter 40.

Terminal illness and death

Humanists do not believe in a God who is involved in human behaviour or way of life. The funeral is therefore a celebration of the life lived and an opportunity to encourage support for the bereaved.

Further reading

Compton's Interactive Encyclopedia (1999) *Enlightenment*. The Learning Company, Cambridge, MA.

Compton's Interactive Encyclopedia (1999) *Humanism*. The Learning Company, Cambridge, MA.

Gilmore MP (1962) *The World of Humanism 1453–1517*. Harper & Row. New York.

Wineriter F (2000) *Living and Dying: Humanism, a rational approach to life and death.* (Text of a lecture presented on 14 September 2000.)

Islam

Origin

Islam is the religion practised by Muslims and is based on the writings of Muhammad, who lived some 1400 years ago. Islam is a whole way of life with legal, moral, political and spiritual guidelines so that every action and thought is guided by complete submission to Allah.

Books and writings

Islam literally means 'submission to God' and is practised by Muslim patients. Islam is based on the teachings of the prophet Muhammad, whom Muslims believe to have received the final revealed word of Allah. Muslims believe that some parts of the divine teachings were revealed in the past through other prophets, including Moses and Jesus Christ, and this final message from Allah is contained in the Koran, which cannot be altered or added to.

Summary of teachings

There are five 'Pillars of Islam' supporting the beliefs and practices of the Islamic faith. These are:

1 **Shahada**: the statement of faith, which includes the statement 'I bear witness that there is no God but Allah and I bear witness that Muhammad is the messenger of Allah'.
2 **Salat**: daily worship: prayers that are recited at dawn, midday, afternoon, evening and night, bowing low down in the direction of Mecca (south-east in Britain). The exact times of sunrise and sunset are used to determine the prayer times. Before praying, one must wash the face, ears, forehead, feet, hands and arms to the elbows. The nose is cleaned by sniffing water and the mouth is rinsed.
3 **Zakat**: charitable giving, which copies the generosity of Allah, partly atones for one's sins and shows practical kindness to the less well off.
4 **Sawm**: fasting, which involves going without food and drink during the hours of daylight in the holy month of Ramadan.
5 **Hajj**: the pilgrimage to Mecca, the birthplace of Muhammad, which healthy Muslim men and women are expected to make at least once in their life.

Islam is a complete way of life and every action and thought should be guided by complete submission to Allah. Friday is the holy day when Muslims visit the mosque.

There is no priest, but the patient might ask for an imam, a learned man of the Muslim faith, to visit. The nearest Islamic centre should be contacted and the details should be available in the telephone directory.

Beliefs and traditions with respect to illness

Muslims do not eat any form of meat that is of pig origin and this includes anything cooked in pig fat. Failure to wash utensils after using them to serve pork renders the food they touch unclean. Meat should be killed according to Muslim law. Some patients might find it preferable for their food to be specially prepared and brought in for them.

Technically, the acutely ill and chronically sick have the option of not fasting during Ramadan but may be reluctant to do this. If the long hours of daylight in the northern hemisphere cause problems, for diabetics for example, the local imam should be contacted so that he can discuss the problem with the patient (and her husband if the patient is a woman).

Drugs and alcohol are expressly forbidden, but allowance may be made for drugs being used for medical purposes, but porcine insulin or other pig products are still forbidden.

Pain is usually seen as the will of Allah and his will should not be resisted. They might wish to have the support of relatives and friends from the local Islamic centre if they feel unable to accept analgesia.

Modesty is of great importance. Women find contact with a male member of staff humiliating and it renders them unclean. Men are dubious about being treated by women and may think of them as of low status for having physical contact with a 'strange man'. Dress is also important and the dress code should be respected.

Muslims have very strong feelings about graft and transplant surgery. Muslims may not receive a transplant, nor can they donate their organs, even within members of their own faith. Tissue grafts of porcine origin are also forbidden.

Terminal illness and death

For the terminally ill Muslim, Ramadan is a final time of putting one's personal spiritual affairs in order. Fasting includes not ingesting anything by mouth, nose, suppository or injection, from dawn to sunset. This may cause problems with symptom control, but many will receive comfort from being able to comply with their religious laws. The use of analgesics with a 24-hour action, offered at a suitable time of day, might afford an acceptable form of pain relief.

Special prayers are recited in Arabic, regardless of nationality. If possible, the patient should join in, facing Mecca. Relatives or Muslims from the local mosque might also wish to recite prayers. The last words a Muslim should utter (always facing Mecca) are the *shahada* – the first words spoken to them at birth: 'There is no God but Allah and Muhammad is his prophet'. Muslims believe that after death, which is seen as a transformation into a new phase of existence, Allah will judge their good and bad deeds, including their charitable giving, and their final utterance of the *shahada* in the hope of mercy in the afterlife.

After death, the body should be washed according to Islamic tradition and wrapped in cloth (men in three pieces of cloth, women in five pieces of cloth). Men must not see or touch a female body after death. Coffins are not acceptable, nor is autopsy. If an autopsy is suggested, the reasons for it being carried out must be discussed with the family.

It is important that burial should take place as quickly as possible, usually within 24 hours. A member of the Muslim community, who will advise the undertaker of the strict code of practice that is followed, usually arranges the funeral. Embalming is not usually carried out and in the UK the body is usually buried, wrapped in a sheet, without a coffin. A coffin may be used for transportation only.

The orientation of the grave is very important, since the body must be placed with the face turned towards Mecca. The surface of the grave must be raised above ground level (which contravenes some cemetery bye-laws), so a special area may be set aside for Muslim burials.

Further reading

Sheikh A and Gatrad AR (2000) *Caring for Muslim Patients*. Radcliffe Medical Press, Oxford.

Judaism

Origin

Judaism is the world's oldest monotheistic religion – one that accepts that there is one God, who created the world and continues to rule over the world.

Books and writings

The word of God was revealed to Moses some 3500 years ago in the Ten Commandments. The first five books of the Old Testament of the Bible are also known as the Torah.

Summary of teachings

Judaism has the central belief that everything is under the control of God. God created man and man's purpose is to recognise and serve God, live a just life, perform good deeds, study the Torah and live accordingly.

The Torah is sometimes referred to as the Written Law, but in addition to this there is the Oral Law contained in the Talmud, the body of Jewish civil and ceremonial law and legend comprising the Mishnah and the Gemara, written between the third and sixth century.

Judaism is therefore sometimes described as a way of life rather than a religion, since it is concerned very much with keeping the Jewish law.

The Sabbath (sundown on Friday to sundown on Saturday) is a very important day for the religious Jew and New Year, the festival of the Passover and the Day of Atonement are also very important days to be observed. To a varying degree, Jews keep the law as laid down in the Ten Commandments.

While Jews believe that the soul is immortal, they concentrate much more on practical issues that make this world a better place in which to live.

Beliefs and traditions with respect to illness

Even the most non-religious Jew retains a very strong sense of the value of human life on the basis that God created man in His own image (Genesis 1:27). This belief in preservation of life is so strong that one may even break certain religious laws in order to preserve a human life. In practice, this means that the terminally ill Jew need not observe festivals or the Sabbath, although many will choose to do so.

An ill Jew will appreciate the lighting of a candle at the beginning of the Sabbath and will also appreciate being given unleavened bread at Passover. (Unleavened bread is relatively easily obtained.) A visit from a Rabbi at Passover will be greatly appreciated.

There are several laws relating to food, the main ones being the forbidding of pork and shellfish and that one should avoid serving meat and milk in the same meal. (This practice relates to the instruction in Exodus 23:19 'Do not cook a young goat in its mother's milk'.) An interval of six hours between consuming meat and drinking milk is usually acceptable.

Terminal illness and death

Food is very important in Jewish life and the family of a terminally ill Jew might bring food in to try to tempt the patient to eat. To the non-Jew, this concern about food may seem inappropriate, but in Judaism it is this life that matters and eating is a sign of holding on to this life and staying in this world. Orthodox Jews do believe in the resurrection of the dead and an afterlife, but the details of what they actually believe vary widely from one person to another.

The importance of the 'here and now' can cause problems for the Jew when dealing with dying patients. Someone who is dying, who will not be in this world for much longer, is not seen as being as important as someone who has a longer life to anticipate. Any form of euthanasia or attempt to shorten life is strongly resisted.

A dying Jew might ask to see the Rabbi. There are no last rites, so a visit is not essential, but if the patient does ask to see the Rabbi, find out whether they are orthodox or non-orthodox Jews and which Rabbi should be called.

After death, it is traditional for the body to be placed on the floor, with the feet towards the door and a burning candle placed near the head. Fellow Jews or family members usually take responsibility for the care of the body, with someone watching over it day and night, reciting psalms continually. This period of watching is not very long, as burial should take place as quickly as possible.

Orthodox Jews are buried in a Jewish cemetery within 24 hours of death. More liberal Jews may allow cremation and the family usually arrange the funeral, which may take place two or three days after the death.

A period of mourning then takes place, initially for seven days, but the full period of mourning is 30 days and after one year the tombstone is consecrated, marking the end of formal mourning.

In the orthodox Jewish religion, post mortem examinations are resisted and giving of organs for transplant is not encouraged. Some more liberal Jews are more relaxed about these laws, so it is worth finding out the wishes of the family.

Further reading

Spitzer J (2003) *Caring for Jewish Patients.* Radcliffe Medical Press, Oxford.

Sikhism

Origin

The term 'Sikh' means 'follower' and the Sikh religion was founded in the fifteenth century by Guru Nanak (1469–1533). ('Guru' means 'spiritual guide'.) Sikhism began in the Punjab and arose when Guru Nanak was examining the differences between Hinduism and Islam. Being unsure which path to follow, he founded a new religion – Sikhism.

The Sikh religion has a strong community aspect and the Sikh temple (gurdwara) is a place of gathering and group activity.

There is no priesthood among Sikhs, with each gurdwara providing the services required in their local Sikh community. Births, marriages, etc. are all celebrated in the gurdwara.

Books and writings

Sikhism has ten Gurus and their collective writings are contained in the *Guru Granth Sahib.* This book is the basis of all Sikh ceremonies and is written in Punjabi. All Sikhs learn to read the Guru Granth Sahib.

Summary of teachings

God created the world and everything in it, but because He is not visible in creation, His will must be made known through the Gurus.

Sikhism is associated with five symbols of faith – 'the five "K"'s'.

1 **Kesh**: uncut hair covered by a turban. The hair is kept in a bun (jura) by both men and women. Women usually don't wear a turban but the men do.
2 **Kanga**: the comb symbolising personal hygiene. A small semi-circular comb is used by both men and women to keep the bun in position. The kanga is a very significant item to a Sikh and if it cannot be in their hair (e.g. if the patient has lost their hair due to chemotherapy), they will want it to be close by and it should never be removed or tidied away.
3 **Kara**: the steel bracelet representing faithfulness to God (originally a protection for the arm carrying the sword). The circular shape represents the unity of God. It should never be removed.
4 **Kirpan**: symbolic dagger symbolising resistance against evil and the Sikh's readiness to fight in self-defence and to protect the poor and oppressed. The size, shape and position of the kirpan and where it is worn all vary. It is important to recognise that the kirpan is worn all the time – at night, in the shower and so on. Do not attempt to remove it on the basis that it may cause injury while sleeping – this causes great distress and may result in the patient losing trust in you and failing to seek help when needed.

If removal is absolutely necessary, the reasons must be fully discussed with the patient and family and the kirpan must be kept within sight of the patient.

5 **Kaccha**: special shorts (underpants) symbolising purity. Traditionally kaccha were knee length, but many Sikhs now wear ordinary underpants instead. As a symbol of modesty and sexual morality, their removal may be strongly resisted. It is common practice for them to be worn in the shower, with a dry pair replacing the wet ones. During practical procedures such as bed-bathing, one leg should always be kept in the kaccha. This is especially important in dying patients.

Beliefs and traditions with respect to illness

Because the gurdwara is the focal point of all activity, any illness which prevents attendance at the gurdwara causes considerable distress. It is common for the gurdwara to arrange for someone to visit and sit with a dying patient.

Traditionally Sikhs rise very early to allow time to wash and spend about two hours in prayer before breakfast. Illness may make this difficult, so the offer of help with washing before prayer will be appreciated. During prayer one should respect the Sikh's privacy and they will be appreciate being left alone.

Terminal illness and death

Sikhs believe that the soul goes through multiple cycles of birth and rebirth, so dying is not frightening. The ultimate aim is to achieve perfection and be reunited with God. How one behaves in this life affects the next life. Fear of dying is therefore likely to be associated with anxiety about what their next life will be like.

After death, the family are usually responsible for looking after the body. Cremation is usual, with the 'five "K"s' being worn on the body. If possible, the cremation should take place within 24 hours of the death. The ashes are usually scattered in a river or the sea.

After the cremation, family and friends will gather at the gurdwara for further prayers before returning home, where it is usual for them to have a shower. The period of mourning lasts for 10–13 days, during which time relatives and friends visit to comfort the bereaved. The home might be used as a temporary temple, with furniture being removed, the floor covered and a canopy erected. If this is not possible, the gurdwara can be used.

At the end of the period of mourning, if the deceased was the head of the family, another ceremony takes place to acknowledge the eldest son as family head. A lamp may be kept lit for several weeks in memory of the deceased person.

Further reading about religious issues with respect to illness

Barnes T (1999) *The Kingfisher Book of Religions*. Kingfisher, London.
Helman C (2000) *Culture, Health and Illness*. Butterworth-Heinemann, Oxford.

Neuberger J (2004) *Caring for Dying People of Different Faiths*. Radcliffe Medical Press, Oxford.

Sampson C (1982) *The Neglected Ethic: cultural and religious factors in the care of patients*. McGraw-Hill, London.

Sheikh A and Gatrad AR (2000) *Caring for Muslim Patients*. Radcliffe Medical Press, Oxford.

Spitzer J (2003) *Caring for Jewish Patients*. Radcliffe Medical Press, Oxford.

Chapter 39

The patient is dying

The doctor says

Unfortunately, I have no choice but to include this chapter because it is something we must face up to.

As carers, it helps if we have some idea about the patient's wishes regarding their funeral arrangements. Someone has to assume responsibility for registering the death. If a will has been made, an executor will have been appointed, but if not, this might be a good time to approach the subject, for it makes things much easier after the patient has passed away.

You might be surprised how often I have been informed, after a patient had died, that nobody in the family knew anything of the patient's wishes regarding their funeral, whether they had made a will and, if so, where it was or which solicitor had helped draw it up. Issues like whether the patient wished to be buried or cremated often had not been discussed and family members sometimes had differing views about what the patient might have wished.

Think

- The person who organises a funeral is usually assumed to be accepting responsibility for the costs. Do you know how these are being met? Make sure there are sufficient funds available to cover the costs of the ceremony and any memorials desired.
- Has the patient made their wishes clear, e.g. is their choice for burial or cremation? Some religions dictate whether burial or cremation is allowed (*see* Chapter 38).
- Who is to be the 'informant' who will register the death? They will need to think about how many copies of the death certificate will be required – e.g. for the bank, or for insurance companies who will not pay out on policies without this confirmation. A fee is payable for these extra copies and the fee increases if copies are requested at a later date and a search is required to find the original entry in the register.

Ask

If the patient is aware that they are dying and has left no instruction about their funeral, you might need to gently explore their wishes in this respect. It's not an easy thing to do, but at the end of the day, it is the patient's wishes that one wishes to fulfil.

If you are not familiar with the patient's personal affairs, you might wish to ask if they have made a will and find out the name of the solicitor who holds the document.

Are there insurance policies and pensions that will need to be dealt with? If so, it might be worthwhile finding out where the patient keeps the papers relating to these and confirming that the monies payable from these have been accounted for in the will. If not, is this a good time to ask the solicitor to make an amendment or redraft the will? Is the patient fit for this?

Note

Make a note of the names of undertakers, solicitors or other persons named by the patient who you may need to contact.

Note the names of people who should conduct the funeral service and make a note of any personal requests – e.g. for scattering of ashes in a favourite place.

Do

After the patient has died, the death certificate can be difficult to understand since it will contain medical terms that are unfamiliar to many people. Ask the doctor who issues the certificate to explain the cause of death, putting the technical language on the form into simpler terms.

Check that there is no reason why you cannot begin the process of arranging the funeral. In other words, confirm that there is no need for a post mortem examination (*see* Chapter 41).

Explore

Find out if there are any special instructions relating to how the body should be handled after the death. This is particularly important in certain religions (*see* Chapter 38).

Does any member of the family have a particular request that they wish to have fulfilled at the time of the funeral – e.g. a special reading or memory that they wish to share?

Look at the section 'More Information' – do you need to confirm any of these details before the patient dies?

More Information

The death must be registered in the area where it occurred.

When registering a death, you need to bring the following documents:

- the death certificate
- the deceased's medical card (if you can find it)
- pension books relating to pensions payable from public funds
- birth and marriage certificates of the deceased.

You also need to be able to tell the registrar:

- the deceased's full name (and maiden name if appropriate)
- the place and date of death
- the usual address where the deceased resided
- the deceased's date and place of birth
- the deceased's occupation and that of their spouse
- the date of birth of their surviving widow(er).

Before a cremation can be arranged, a second independent doctor must examine the body of the deceased and issue a further certificate. You do not have to arrange this, the doctor who issued the death certificate will do that, but you should be aware that it is routine practice and implies no concern or doubt about the cause of death. The need for a second doctor to examine the body should not cause any delay in making the funeral arrangements.

Patients who have suffered from cancer cannot usually have their organs used for transplants. One possible exception is the use of the corneas of the eyes. In general, the tissues being donated must be removed very quickly – 30 minutes in the case of internal organs and 24 hours in the case of corneas. If organ donation was the patient's wish, it may not be possible due to the nature of their illness. There are obvious time-related problems associated with a death at home, but if you do wish to explore the donation of corneas, contact your nearest eye hospital without delay.

Further reading

Weller S (1999) *Guide to Funerals and Bereavement* (*The Daily Telegraph* lifeplanner). Kogan Page, London.

Chapter 40

Euthanasia, advance directives and related topics

The doctor says

This is a complicated subject and one in which the law and public attitudes are changing. I have tried to reflect a variety of current opinions by quoting several points of view, mostly published in the months before this book went to press. My own personal view is that euthanasia is morally wrong, and that with good palliative care one should not need to ask for an early death. I also am concerned that a premature death, at the hand of a third person and at a time of their choice, can deprive the patient of the opportunity to make peace with God before dying.

Here we will think about three issues – euthanasia, advance directives and instructions not to resuscitate the patient.

Euthanasia

Euthanasia is an act intended to shorten life. It is classified as follows.

- Voluntary euthanasia is carried out at the specific request of a competent patient.
- Involuntary euthanasia is carried out without the request of a competent patient.
- Non-voluntary euthanasia is carried out when the patient is incapable of giving meaningful consent.

At the time of writing, all forms of euthanasia are criminal acts in the UK. Euthanasia is legal in some countries (e.g. Holland) and the Dutch Justice Minister has recently ruled that dementia is a valid reason for euthanasia. A report in *Image News* (July 2004 edition) states that 'the British Government is against active euthanasia but supports changing the law to allow euthanasia by neglect'.[1] The word 'neglect' here refers to acts such as withholding food and fluids from patients, thus hastening their death.

Professor Tim Maughan[2] of the University of Wales College of Medicine points out that those in favour of euthanasia might argue on grounds of:

- compassion, saying that a death with dignity is preferable to suffering
- autonomy, arguing for the 'right to die'
- economics, because keeping people alive is expensive.

He also outlines the other points of view, namely that euthanasia is:

- unnecessary, because symptoms can usually be effectively controlled
- dangerous, because the terminally ill patient usually is vulnerable and may be poorly informed of the symptom control measures available
- regarded as morally wrong by most religious faiths and forbidden by all traditional codes of medical ethics.

Living wills (advance directives)

While a will is usually a document dealing one's affairs regarding the funeral and the distribution of one's estate after death, you should be aware of the concept of the 'living will'.

Living wills or 'advance directives' are the wishes of a person, recorded and witnessed at a time when they are in good health and of sound mind.

Living wills are frequently assumed only to instruct that no attempt should be made to resuscitate the patient in the event of illness such that they are deprived of quality of life and become a burden on others for their care.

Dr Michael Irwin,[3] a former Vice Chairman of the Voluntary Euthanasia Society, points out that an advance directive can equally state that a person wishes to be kept alive as long as possible and gives consent to all medical procedures necessary. A third type of living will may only give consent to measures directed at symptom control and freedom from pain.

Depending on its content, the document may have no legal status and may in fact request an action that is illegal in the UK.

This is an area where things are changing and if the patient has written an advance directive, or is thinking of doing so, they must seek expert legal and medical advice. You need to be aware of the patient's wishes, but you may feel unable to carry them out, even if they are legal.

'Do not resuscitate'

The instruction 'do not resuscitate' may be considered acceptable in the event of a sudden collapse when it is thought likely that attempts to resuscitate the patient will be unsuccessful or that they might only survive for a very short time.

The British Medical Association and the Royal College of Nursing guidelines[4] on 'Do Not Resuscitate (DNR) Statements' include the following: 'It is appropriate to consider a DNR decision . . . where the patient's condition indicates that effective cardiopulmonary resuscitation is unlikely to be successful . . .'

A report of the views of a group of oncology nurses[5] showed that they felt that resuscitation might be inappropriate if:

- it was unlikely to be successful
- it was not in agreement with the expressed wishes of a competent patient
- a valid advance directive refused resuscitation
- successful resuscitation would result only in a poor quality of life.

This is a very difficult subject to think about and one that both the patient and their carers need to discuss. The patient must ensure that everyone understands their wishes in this respect.

Basically, the thought is that if one is dying of cancer, a sudden event such as a heart attack could be a quicker and easier release for the patient. It is hard for the family and those who have cared for the patient not to feel that they should have tried some form of resuscitation.

Think

- Why is the patient raising this topic now?
- Is the patient asking for euthanasia, or for treatment to be discontinued – 'allowing nature to take its course'?
- Is the patient actually expressing a perceived lack of physical, emotional or spiritual support?
- Has the patient expressed any fear of the process of dying?
- Is someone or something pressurising the patient to consider euthanasia?
- Do you think the patient might feel that they are a burden on their family or carers?
- Do you think the patient might be depressed? (*See* Chapter 18.)
- Could the patient be feeling a loss of their personal dignity?

You also need to think about the doctors and nurses who are caring for the patient. Think about:

- their legal position
- their ethical position.

They will remind the patient and you of their legal position if the subject of euthanasia is raised. As the law stands now, breach of the law carries an automatic erasure from the General Medical Council register and the register of nurses and the automatic loss of a job for the doctor and nurse.

Ask

- If you think the patient is afraid of the process of dying, talk to the doctor or nurse about this. It is a common fear and their anxieties may be unfounded.
- If the patient is asking about euthanasia, you can discuss this confidentially with the staff. They will be able to offer you appropriate advice and support. Hospices and palliative care units specialise in controlling symptoms and allowing patients to die with dignity in peaceful surroundings.
- If the patient admits to feeling that they have become a burden on their family or carers, discuss this with the patient, the family and the nurse and doctor. Perhaps the patient is aware that you need a break and a respite admission in the hospice may be a realistic option. Do not feel guilty for agreeing to an admission to give you a break. Some carers will not admit to needing to 'recharge their batteries' but nobody should be expected to work without a short holiday, allowing them to come back refreshed.

- Encourage the patient to speak to a minister or religious adviser if they have expressed anxiety or feel that they are not prepared for dying and need to discuss religious and spiritual matters (*see* Chapter 38).

Note

If the patient has mentioned any specific requests about what should happen after their death, it might help for you to write these down, keep the instructions safe and ensure that they are given to the person who is responsible for arranging the funeral.

If there any specific religious or cultural requirements regarding the handling of the patient's body after death, make sure that hospital staff are aware of these instructions and that the person who is responsible for arranging the funeral also knows of these requirements.

Do

If you suspect that the patient is depressed, encourage them to discuss this with the doctor or nurse.

If the patient has made any specific requests, e.g. an advance directive or a request not to resuscitate, make sure that an independent person is aware of these wishes and, if possible, get these requests in writing and get the statement signed by a reliable witness.

Explore

The law and ethical views concerning euthanasia and the related issue of advance directives are very complex. You might wish to think about these situations.

- Is withdrawing or not starting a futile treatment – e.g. antibiotics in terminal bronchopneumonia – euthanasia or is it the most appropriate and ethical way to manage a patient's care?
- Are food and fluids delivered by tube 'treatment'?

The law in many countries is changing and as new cases come before the courts, our laws may change too.

More Information

A report in the *British Medical Journal*[6] showed that 80% of patients questioned wished to die with their symptoms relieved.

Another report, also in the *British Medical Journal*,[7] points out that good symptom control at the end of life might lead to fewer requests for euthanasia.

Palliative care is about trying to maximise quality of life without necessarily prolonging life. The staff will do their utmost to alleviate the patient's distressing symptoms – physical, social, emotional and spiritual.

References

1 *Image News*, July 2004. Published by IMAGE, Coverdale Centre, Ardwick, Manchester M12 4FG.
2 Maughan T (2003) *Euthanasia*. CMF Files number 23. Published by Christian Medical Fellowship, 157 Waterloo Road, London SE1 8XN.
3 Irwin M (2003) A new kind of living will. *Journal of the Royal Society of Medicine.* **96**: 411.
4 British Medical Association Resuscitation Council (UK) and Royal College of Nursing (2001) *Decisions Relating to Cardiopulmonary Resuscitation.* BMA, London.
5 Bass M (2003) Oncology nurses' perceptions of their role in resuscitation decisions. *Professional Nurse.* **18**(12): 710–13.
6 Clark J (2003) Freedom from unpleasant symptoms is essential for a good death. *BMJ.* **327**: 180.
7 Mak YYW, Elwyn G and Finlay IG (2003) Patients' voices are needed in debates on euthanasia. *BMJ.* **327**: 213–15.

Chapter 41

A further examination of the body has been ordered

Having to face the trauma of a patient dying is bad enough, but to have to agree to an autopsy is even more difficult.

There are two basic questions that we need to ask. These are:

- When is a further examination of the body necessary?
- Why is a further examination of the body necessary?

We will now look at these in turn.

When is a further examination of the body necessary?

Most countries have a legal procedure for the investigation of deaths for which the cause is not precisely known. The coroner, who is usually either a lawyer or a doctor, is employed to enquire into various types of deaths at the request of a doctor, the police and, occasionally, the public, where certain facts necessary for the certification of the death are not known. These include the following circumstances:

- During their final illness, the deceased person was not attended by any doctor.
- The deceased was not seen by a doctor in the 14 days before their death.
- The cause of death is uncertain.
- The death may be due to industrial disease, e.g. exposure to asbestos.
- The death occurred during an operation or before recovery from the anaesthetic.
- The death may be due to poisoning.
- The death may be due to unnatural causes.
- The death occurred in suspicious circumstances.

In certain areas of Wales all deaths occurring in miners are subject to an autopsy to determine whether industrial factors played a part.

Why is a further examination of the body necessary?

We can break this answer into three basic parts, addressing the people who might benefit from such a procedure.

The bereaved relatives

- The actual cause of death is established in those situations where it was previously not certain.

- You can hopefully be assured that the disease could not have been discovered earlier and that nothing was missed that should have been detected at an earlier stage.
- If the disease was inherited or could be linked to a genetic cause, you will be aware and have an opportunity to have the appropriate checks made on members of the family who could be at risk.
- Any undiagnosed infections, e.g. tuberculosis, will be detected and appropriate checks can be made to see that you and others are not infected.

The medical profession

- In those cases where there was a delay in detecting the nature of the illness or where a wrong diagnosis was made, the information gained will be used to educate and inform, hopefully preventing this happening to another patient.
- Unusual presentations of disease are recorded and this information is used to teach doctors and alert them to the possibility of similar situations. This information is completely anonymous and individuals cannot be identified.
- The effects of treatment can be assessed and any findings be made known so that, in combination with other research, treatments can be made even more effective.

Society

- Medical knowledge is improved and extended. This will not help the patient, but they will be helping others.

Sometimes, when a doctor is unsure about the exact cause of death, they might refer the matter to the coroner for further advice. The two common outcomes are that either:

1 the coroner is satisfied, after a full discussion, that there is no need for an autopsy and the doctor can issue the death certificate, allowing arrangements for the funeral to proceed

or:

2 the coroner may request a further examination of the body. If this shows that the death is due to natural causes, the coroner issues the death certificate allowing the family to arrange the funeral.

Chapter 42

Coping with bereavement

The doctor says

Bereavement and loss affect everyone differently and there is no 'right' or 'wrong' way to cope with the loss of a loved one. There have been many studies carried out to examine how people cope with bereavement and this section outlines what might happen in your case. You might not experience some of these feelings and the times suggested are averages, which can vary enormously. One popular teaching about bereavement is to consider the following four 'stages'.

Stage 1: Shock and disbelief

This stage may last up to two weeks and you could experience a lack of strength and appetite, choking sensations and breathlessness. These physical reactions may come in waves.

It can be difficult at this stage to accept the reality of the death and you may feel numb and detached from the events that have so recently affected you.

Stage 2: Awareness develops

Physically, you may feel a lack of energy and symptoms of stress.
Emotionally, there may be a variety of reactions:

- crying
- hearing the deceased person's voice
- a desire to search for the deceased person who is 'missing'
- guilt
- anger – against doctors or the hospital, other members of the family, God or the deceased person for dying.

Stage 3: Depression

You may feel a lack of interest in your own life and the lives of others. Life may seem lacking in purpose.

Stage 4: Resolution

Gradually you recognise that you will be able to cope and enjoy life again in a new way without experiencing feelings of disloyalty towards the deceased. This may take up to 1–2 years.

You might feel guilty for redeveloping your social life, especially if you were caring for the patient for a long time and gave up many of your own leisure and pleasure interests to make time for the patient and their care.

Meeting old friends can be difficult. It won't be the same if you and the patient usually met friends together as a couple. Meeting them alone is quite different.

Feelings of guilt about going on holiday are also common and are normal, but you are allowed to rebuild your life.

Think

At the time a death occurs, there are many things going on and it may be after the funeral that you have questions in your mind. Here are some of the things that you might wish to think about.

Did you understand the exact cause of death? Sometimes the medical terminology used on death certificates seems to give a different reason for the cause of death from what you understood it to be. A death certificate is a legal document, so the doctor must use the correct medical terms. These are often unfamiliar and can be misunderstood. Don't be afraid to ask for clarification about anything that is causing you concern. Do not sit worrying that there might have been something else that you or someone else could have done. It's a common worry and is almost always unfounded.

Are there any aspects of the final care given that you are unsure about?

Did the patient have children in the family who might need support at this difficult time?

Ask

If there is anything in the death certificate that you are unsure about, ask for an explanation about the exact cause of death.

If you have concerns over any aspect of the care given in the patient's final illness, it is easiest to resolve this now. In my 25 years in medicine, inferior quality of care is rarely the case but an explanation of what was being done, and why, could have saved much unnecessary anxiety.

Note

Make a note of the names of people or organisations that might offer help and support to you during this difficult time. There may be a local group based at the hospital or hospice or you might wish to speak to someone in a national organisation such as Cruse.

Do ✔

Look after yourself. It is very common for a bereaved person to not wish to eat, to sleep poorly and sometimes lose interest in oneself. Try to establish a routine in your life which includes a regular bedtime. It is important to try and avoid using sleeping tablets if at all possible. Sleeping tablets and tranquillisers are rarely helpful and when they are necessary their use should be for as short a time as possible.

If the patient's illness was a long one, it is probably some time since you have thought about your own health and welfare. If you have any concerns about your own health (which is not uncommon at this time), see your doctor.

Explore

When you feel that the time is right, explore a new hobby or interest. You may feel guilty about doing so, but you are allowed to 'move on' and take time for yourself and time to rebuild your life.

More Information

Coping with your loss should become easier with the passage of time but there are times when that can be particularly difficult. These include:

- birthdays
- Christmas
- holidays
- special family events – e.g. a wedding with one parent missing
- the first anniversary of the death
- wedding anniversaries.

It might help for you to arrange to be with family or close friends at these difficult times, especially in the first year.

Further reading

Catlett E (2000) *When Someone Dies*. Elliot Right Way Books, Kingswood, Surrey.
Weller S (1999) *The Daily Telegraph Guide to Funerals and Bereavement*. Kogan Page, London.

Appendices

The following pages may be photocopied so that you can use them
as often as you need to.

Glossary of medical words

Acupressure
An ancient Chinese therapy involving pressure applied over various points on the body instead of the needles used in acupuncture.

Acupuncture
An ancient Chinese therapy involving the insertion of fine needles at various points on the body.

Advance directive
See *living will*.

Anaemia
Literally means 'bloodless'. The condition of having less red blood cells than normal due to blood loss, lack of iron in the diet, or myelosuppression due to treatment for cancer.

Aromatherapy
A treatment involving the use of plant essential oils combined with gentle massage. The oils used by professional aromatherapists are highly concentrated and must only be used by trained staff. They are much purer and more highly concentrated than the cheap oils and burners sold in high street shops.

Autopsy
An examination of the organs of a dead body to determine the cause of death or to study the changes caused by disease.

Bronchoscope
A rigid or flexible endoscope for inspecting the interior of the air passages to your lung, either for diagnostic purposes (e.g. biopsy) or for the removal of foreign bodies.

Bronchoscopy
Inspection of the interior of the air passages to your lungs through a bronchoscope.

Chemotherapy
The use of drugs to kill cancer cells. These are often given by injection or a drip into your veins, but may be given as tablets.

Denial
An unconscious defence mechanism used to allay anxiety by denying the existence of important conflicts or troublesome thoughts.

DNR
A short form of 'Do Not Resuscitate', a statement that might be written on the notes, indicating an agreement that the patient's condition indicates that effective cardiopulmonary resuscitation is unlikely to be successful.

Edema
See *oedema*.

Endoscope
A flexible instrument for the examination of the interior of a hollow part of the body, e.g. the bowel. The endoscope may carry a small camera and can also be used for taking small samples for further examination.

Endoscopy	Examination of the interior of a hollow part of the body e.g. gullet or bowel, by means of an endoscope.
Euthanasia	The intentional putting to death of a person with an incurable or painful disease, intended as an act of mercy.
Fistula	An abnormal passage from one surface to another surface – opening from both sides (compare *sinus*).
Fungating	Growing exuberantly like a fungus or spongy growth.
Hickman line	A cannula (a fine polythene tube) inserted into the veins in the neck and ending up in the large blood vessels near the heart. It can be used to take blood samples, give drugs and for feeding or giving fluids in a seriously ill patient.
Homoeopathy (sometimes spelled homeopathy)	A system of therapy, 'law of similia' (likes are cured by likes), which holds that a medicinal substance that can evoke certain symptoms in healthy individuals may be effective in the treatment of illnesses having symptoms closely resembling those produced by the substance.
Hydrotherapy	The use of water, often in a specially designed swimming pool, to assist with exercise and to strengthen weak muscles.
Jaundice	A yellowish staining of the eyes and skin, and associated with dark urine due to increased amounts of bile pigments in the blood.
Living will	Also called an 'advance directive', these are the wishes of a person, recorded and witnessed at a time when they are in good health and of sound mind. The living will normally instructs that no attempt should be made to resuscitate the patient in the event of illness such that they are deprived of quality of life and become a burden on others for their care. Depending on its content, the document may have no legal status, or may even request an act that is currently illegal in the UK.
Lymph	A clear, transparent, sometimes faintly yellow fluid that is collected from the tissues throughout the body, flows in the lymphatic vessels (through the lymph nodes), and is eventually added to the venous blood circulation.
Lymphoedema	Swelling (often of an arm or leg) as a result of obstruction of lymphatic vessels or lymph nodes and the accumulation of large amounts of lymph in the affected region.
Myelosuppression	A reduction in the normal function of your bone marrow. The bone marrow makes blood cells – red cells to carry oxygen, white cells to help fight infection.

Myelosuppression is a side effect of many cancer treatments and results in reduced resistance to disease and can result in anaemia and subsequent shortness of breath.

Obturator A specially designed denture used to close an opening in the roof of the mouth after surgery.

Oedema (edema in American texts) An accumulation of an excessive amount of watery fluid in the tissues. This is usually seen as swollen ankles.

Pain assessment tools These are a variety of numeric, verbal and visual scales designed to help patients record the severity of their pain. To document the effect of any change in the patient's medication, the assessment should be carried out on a regular basis until pain is controlled.

Palliative treatment Treatment intended to relieve symptoms without curing the underlying disease.

Phantom limb The sensation that an amputated limb is still present, often associated with painful abnormal sensations such as burning, pricking, tickling or tingling.

PICC line 'PICC' is a short form of 'peripherally inserted central catheter'. These are fine tubes inserted into a vein and they are used to give drugs and to feed the patient if necessary. They can be left in place for some time and avoid the need for repeated puncturing of veins to obtain blood samples.

Prognosis A forecast of the probable course and/or outcome of a disease.

Radiotherapy The use of high energy X-rays to kill cancer cells. The patient must lie very still on a table like an X-ray table. Treatment sessions usually last for a couple of minutes but may take several minutes to set up while patients are positioned. The radiotherapy beam must be very accurately focused and positioned, so small tattoo marks may be made on the skin or mouldings may be made to ensure that the treatment positions are exactly reproduced at each treatment session.

Sinus A cavity or hollow space. A sinus is a blind cul-de-sac that opens to one surface only (compare *fistula*).

Tenesmus An urgent desire to evacuate the bowel or bladder, involuntary straining, and the passage of little faecal matter or urine.

Tumour The word 'tumour' literally means any kind of abnormal lump or growth, which may be benign (non-cancerous) or malignant (cancer) but in this book it refers specifically to a cancerous growth.

Patient's pain record

If the patient is not able to report their symptoms effectively, you may wish to use this diagram to mark where the patient has pain. If the patient has more than one pain, mark each one. You may find it helpful to use a different colour of pen for each pain and use the same colour for any description or notes you wish to record about each of the pains.

If the patient cannot speak, mark the places where they seem to be sore when touched.

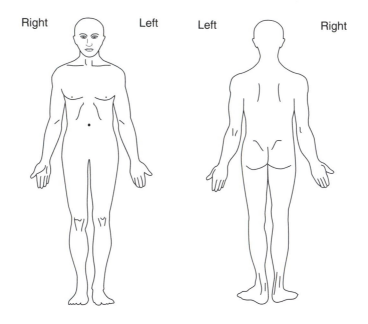

Use these diagrams to mark:

- where the patient's pain is and where it goes
- the date on which this information was recorded
- a brief description of each pain.

Medication chart

Regular medications

Name of medication and what it's for	Times to be taken						
	6am	8am	10am	12md	2pm	6pm	10pm

Medications to be given if needed

Name of medication and what it's for	How often can I give it per 24 hours?	Tell the doctor or nurse if . . .

Useful organisations

Acupuncturists

British Acupuncture Council
Tel: 020 8735 0400
Website: www.acupuncture.org.uk

Aromatherapy

Aromatherapy Organisations Council
PO Box 19834
London SE25 6WF
Tel: 020 8251 7912 (10am–2pm)
Provides a list of qualified practitioners in your area

Bereavement

Cruse Bereavement Care
Cruse House
126 Sheen Road
Richmond
Surrey TW9 1UR
Helpline: 0870 167 1677
All types of bereavement counselling and a range of publications

National Association of Bereavement Services
2nd Floor
4 Pinchin Street
London E1 1SA
Helpline: 020 7709 9090
Keeps a nationwide directory of bereavement and loss services and has local groups for various different religions and races. Staffed by bereavement counsellors

The Compassionate Friends
53 North Street
Bristol BS3 1EN
Helpline: 0117 953 9639
A nationwide organisation offering support to parents and families after the death of a child

Winston's Wish
Clara Burgess Centre
Gloucester Royal Hospital
Great Western Road
Gloucester GL50 3AW
Helpline: 0845 203 0405
Provides a range of services for bereaved children and their families

Bristol Cancer Help Centre	Grove House Cornwallis Grove Bristol BS8 4PG Information line: 0117 980 0500 *Provides a holistic approach to complementary care for cancer patients*
CancerBACUP	3 Bath Place Rivington Street London EC2A 3JR Tel: 020 7696 9003 Website: www.cancerbacup.org.uk *Support and publications for patients, relatives and professionals in a variety of languages*
Cancer Care	Sue Ryder Care Healthcare Services PO Box 5044 Ashby de la Zouch Leicestershire LE65 1ZP Tel: 01332 694800 *Homes specialising in cancer care and visiting nurses to care for patients in their own homes* Marie Curie Cancer Care 89 Albert Embankment London SE1 7TP Tel: 020 7599 7777 *(Scotland)* 29A Albany Street Edinburgh EH1 3QN Tel: 0131 456 3700 *Home nursing service for day and night care*
Carers National Association	20–25 Glasshouse Yard London EC1A 4JS *(Scotland)* 3rd Floor 162 Buchanan Street Glasgow G1 2LL *Information and advice for carers. Can advise you of carers' groups in your area*
Children	Sargent Cancer Care for Children Griffin House 161 Hammersmith Road London W6 8SG Tel: 020 8752 2800 *Can provide cash grants for parents of children with cancer to help with costs of clothing, travel, equipment, etc.*

Chiropractic	Chiropractic Patients' Association (CPA) Tel: 01722 415 027 Website: www.chiropractic.uk *The General Chiropractic Council can help you find a chiropractor in your area* Tel: 0845 601 1796 Website: www.gcc.uk.org
Counselling	British Association for Counselling and Psychotherapy 1 Regent Place Rugby Warwickshire CV21 2PJ Tel: 0870 443 5252 *Publishes a directory of counsellors in the UK*
DVLA	*To check about notifiable medical conditions and see updated information from DVLA, look at their website www.dvla.gov.uk/drivers/dmed1*
Herbal practitioners	British Herbal Medicine Association Sun House Church Street Stroud Gloucestershire GL5 1JL Tel: 01453 751389 *Provides an information service and list of qualified herbal practitioners*
Homoeopathy	The Faculty of Homoeopathy and British Homoeopathic Association Tel: 0870 444 3955 *Provides details of doctors and dentists who practise homoeopathy*
Hospices	Hospice Information Service St Christopher's Hospice 51–59 Lawrie Park Road London SE26 6DZ Tel: 020 8778 9252 *Information about hospices and hospice care*
Institute for Complementary Medicine	PO Box 194 London SE16 1QZ *Send a SAE with two loose stamps for information*
Ireland – health advice	*Irishhealth. Free advice and information online and articles and resources on health in Ireland. All medical content is approved by Irish healthcare professionals* Website: www.irishhealth.com
Lloyds pharmacy	*Produce an Independent Living Catalogue of products to help people maintain an active and healthy lifestyle*

Macmillan Cancerline	Tel: 0808 808 2020 (Monday–Friday, 9am–5pm)
	Advice and information on all aspects of cancer
Macmillan Cancer Relief Information Line	Tel: 0845 601 6161
Reflexologists	Association of Reflexologists
	27 Old Gloucester Street
	London WC1N 3XX
	Tel: 0870 567 3320
	Provides a list of qualified practitioners in your area
St John Ambulance	Check telephone directory for local offices
	Advice about getting equipment on loan
Tak Tent Cancer Support Scotland	Tel: 0141 211 0122
	Information and support group network across Scotland
Tenovus Cancer Information Centre	Tel: 029 2019 6100
	A range of support services for people in Wales (available in English and Welsh)

Who's who?

General practitioner
Dr _____
Address _____
_____
Telephone (normal hours) _____
Telephone (outwith normal hours) _____

Community nurse
Name _____
Address _____
_____
Telephone (normal hours) _____
Telephone (outwith normal hours) _____

Consultant (Specialist in   )
Dr _____
Hospital address _____
Telephone _____ extension number _____
Patient's hospital number _____

Consultant (Specialist in   )
Dr _____
Hospital address _____
Telephone _____ extension number _____
Patient's hospital number _____

Consultant (Specialist in) _____
Dr _____
Hospital address _____
Telephone _____ extension number _____
Patient's hospital number _____

Consultant (Specialist in   )
Dr _____
Hospital address _____
Telephone _____ extension number _____
Patient's hospital number _____

Clinical nurse specialist (specialising in   )
Name _____
Telephone _____ extension number _____ pager _____

Clinical nurse specialist (specialising in   )
Name _____
Telephone _____ extension number _____ pager _____

Clinical nurse specialist (specialising in   )
Name _____
Telephone _____ extension number _____ pager _____

Macmillan nurse
Name _____
Telephone _____ extension number _____

Marie Curie nurse
Name _____
Telephone _____ extension number _____

Social worker _____
Name _____
Telephone _____ extension number _____

Bereavement counsellor
Name _____
Telephone _____ extension number _____

Others
Name _____ Professional role _____
Telephone _____ extension number _____

Name _____ Professional role _____
Telephone _____ extension number _____

Name _____ Professional role _____
Telephone _____ extension number _____

Name _____ Professional role _____
Telephone _____ extension number _____

Name _____ Professional role _____
Telephone _____ extension number _____

Index

3